A 90 Day Challenge for Husbands and Wives to Exercise Together:

A Step by Step Guide on How to Get This Done

Written By: Elizabeth Tayem and Eric Tangumonkem

Table of Contents

Introduction

Many married couples find it difficult to exercise because they do not have a road map. In our book titled, "The Secret to Husbands and wives exercising together we shared our own frustrations, failures and eventual victory after more than a decade of trying to exercise together. We strongly believe that part of the reason we failed is because we were not having a road map. The desire to take care of our health through exercise was there and we on many occasions went out and tried unsuccessfully to exercise, but the road was filled with some many "landmines" and we kept stepping on them. For example, we argued a lot and got angry at each other and this negative energy sabotaged our exercise effort and we gave up. We could have avoided these "landmines and many other pitfalls if we have a roadmap.

This roadmap is a result of close to a decade of exercising together and regularly as husband and wife. Our aha moment was precipitated by a near death experience my wife went through and after that we decided to take exercise more seriously. The gravity of the situation galvanized us to come up with a very strong "WHY" to exercise as a couple. Our why is so strong that it has enabled us to overcome hot, cold weather and all sorts of condition to exercise. Our goal was to stay healthy, but it turned out that our marriage was going to benefit tremendously from exercising regularly.

That is why we are putting this resource to help you learn how to use one stone and shoot two birds. In other words, you will be maximizing your time by exercising together for the sake of your health and your marriage. The 30 to 45 minutes that you will spend together exercising as husband and wife is going to have a multiplier effect on your heath, quality of sex, communication, increase your intimacy and save you tons of money. You cannot go wrong exercising together as a couple. There are too many benefits that we do not have room here to enumerate. Seeing is believing and when you go through these 90 days exercise challenge you will see firsthand the positive effect exercising regularly will have on the quality of your communication, sex and intimacy. Above all your health is going to improve and if you are already in good health, you will get into top health.

There is no substitute to exercising together if you want a robust, vital, and strong lasting marriage. While Viagra and other drugs have their place in improving and enhancing libido, exercising regularly has far more benefits and it is more holistic. If you and your husband or wife already exercise regularly but separately, we are suggesting and encouraging both of you to start exercising together. There is a lot of benefits exercising, but it is even more beneficial exercising together and regularly.

He purposes of this manual is to take out the guess work and give you something that works. Your part is to follow the instructions; take action and you will have results. It is going to require sacrifice, compromise, dying to self and letting love to take over. This is a challenging call, but we know since you are reading this manual you have what it takes to turn your marriage around. This journey is not for the faint hearted, and you are bold, assertive focused and determined. Therefore, nothing is going to stop you. This is an action book and there is no room for theories. If you want to change you must change something and here is an excellent opportunity to do that.

We are aware of the difficulties, challenges, and typical excuses many couples have to overcome to make this work. That is why this roadmap us designed in a way that it is easy to use and follow and apply. We strong suggest that you and your husband or wife follow the instruction in this manual closely. We will be available during these 90 days to answer your questions, concerns or just celebrate your victories with you. The best way to contact us with you questions, concerns and success stories is through 90daysexercisechallenge@gmail.com

The emphasis here are on doing and we hope that you are going to commit for the next 90 days to do all it is going to take to turn your marriage around and position it to flourish for a long time.

First Things First

Before we embark on this challenge it is important to do some housekeeping, because it will determine how successful you are going to be. It is going to be challenging, but you will do great as long as you follow the ground rules that we are going to lay down. Most of what we are going to be talking about is information that you already know, and we will just be helping organize it in a way that makes sense. There is a great potential for conflict, and we must be careful how we proceed on this journey. Part of the reason you have not been able to exercise together as husband and wife may be due to the fact that you are avoiding having conflicts with each other. In the short run this makes sense, but the future of your marriage is being undermined. Therefore, it is imperative for take some concerted effort.

1) Do a Medical Checkup

You need to establish the baseline of your health so that you will have something to gauge your progress against. Facts do not lie and the only way to truly know the state of your health is to get a medical professional to check you. Instead of fighting over if you should exercise or not or insisting that you are set in your ways and there is no need to change, your medical results and the advice of the doctor will guide you on what to do. It is crucial for you to know the following, your vital signs (blood pressure, heart rate, respiratory rate), blood sugar, cholesterol, etc.

If you cannot afford to get an annual physical done or live where there is no doctor, this should not prevent you from doing this challenge. Doing the medical exam is crucial but it is not mandatory if you cannot afford it. Therefore, do not use the absence of a doctor as an excuse to back out of this challenge.

2) Calculate Your Body Mass Index (BMI)

Many people do not like to talk about their weight and get overly defense about it. Your feelings or what you think about your weight does not count. If you want to get your health back, you have to be willing to do something else and make the necessary changes. One way is by calculating your BMI and it will let you know where you are for numbers do not lie. Here is the formula to calculate the BMI. The formula is BMI = P/W^2 where, P your weight in pounds and W^2 is your height in feet squared.

BMI Categories:
- Underweight = <18.5
- Normal weight = 18.5–24.9
- Overweight = 25–29.9
- Obesity = BMI of 30 or greater

You and your husband or wife should also take your weight, measure your height, and calculate your Body Mass Index (BMI).

My Weight is:

_____

_____

My Height is:

_____

_____

My BMI is:

_____

_____

3) Come Up with Your Why

A strong why is imperative for you to succeed on this 90-day challenge. Without a good why and solid goals you are not going to make it, no matter how much you want it or desire it. If you had read our book titled. "Couples exercising together" We discussed at length on the importance of having a strong why. This has to be something that you and your husband or wife agree on. Your why must be bigger than both of you. In other words, you have to think about the other couples and people that will benefit from your success. It is not always about us, but about others. That is why we are blessed to be a blessing. This does not mean that you will lose anything if you factor other people into your why. Instead you will win more when you understand and operate by the law of being blessed to be a blessing. These questions may help you as you think about your why. How important is your marriage to you? What are you willing to sacrifice to have a vibrant, exciting, and rewarding marriage? What are some of the things that are hampering intimacy in your marriage? On the scale of 1 to 10 how can your rank the quality of your marriage? If your score is below 7 do you like where you are? If there was more to be experienced in marriage will you do what it takes to tap into it?

When you and your husband or wife come up with your why write here and also write in and place it on your bathroom mirror or anywhere in the house where you can see it each day. You will be required to read it each morning during the 90-day challenge. The purpose is to program your why in your subconscious mind. When you successfully program your why, it will take a life of its own and propel you to success.

Our why is

_____

_____

_____

_____

_____

4) Set Goals

If you do not know where you are going you are never going to know when you arrive. There is a lot that has been written about **SMART** goals.

Specific: You have to be specific as possible. For example, we are going to lose 10 pounds.

Measurable: When you get on the scale and measure yourself you will know how well you are doing with your goal of losing 10 pounds.

Achievable: It will be unwise to set a goal that cannot be achieved. If you have never ran a mile you cannot say you are going to run 100 on the first run. Is losing 10 pounds achievable? Yes!

Relevant: Your why is at the heart of every goal that you will set, for it gives it relevance. Why are you losing 10 pounds is more extremely important? There is an enormous financial, and health benefits associated with exercising.

Time-bound: Most goals are never achieved because there is no deadline associated with the goal. You do not have an entire lifetime to achieve your goals. In this case you have 90 days to achieve these goals you are going to set. Can you lose 10 pounds in 90 days? Here is an example of a SMART goal. *"I am going to lose 10 pounds within 90 days."*

You are going to come up with 5 goals that you will like to achieve as a couple during these 90 days. Remember that we are focusing on the positive impact exercise can have on your marriage in the area of money, sex, and communication. Let your goals reflect these three areas. You should have two goals in each category, but if you think some areas need more help, you need at least one goal from each area.

Goal #1

_____

_____

_____

Goal #2

_____

_____

_____

Goal #3

_____

_____

_____

Goal #4

_____

_____

_____

Goal #5

_____

_____

_____

Goal #6

_____

_____

_____

5) Decide When to Exercise

Some people say they can only exercise in the morning and some in the evening. It is going to be challenging to select time of day that both you and your husband or wife will exercise together, because you maybe on totally different clocks. We are leaving it up to you to decide how to make this happen, because you must figure out how both of you will exercise. There is no excuse that is good enough for you and your husband not to exercise together regularly. Now is the opportunity to learn how to compromise and how to give and take. You might have been used to "my way our we go our separate ways" this is an easy way, but it undermines your marriage in the long run. Now is the time for our way is the only way. Somehow you will agree either to exercise in the morning or evening or midnight. The key is that both of you have to go out together. We will suggest that exercising first thing in the morning is one of the best things you can ever do for your marriage. Because it is easier to get it out of your way when you get up and avoid the tiredness that may creep in during the day from preventing you from going out to exercise. That said it is ultimate; left up to both of you to select what time of the day that will work best for you. What is more important is that both of you actually go out together and exercise.

6) Choose Where to Exercise

There are many different places for both of you to exercise together and this will be influenced by what part of the world you live in. We say so because weather is a big factor in determine if you are going to exercise outdoors or indoors. But you should not allow the weather to prevent you from doing what is good for you, your health, and your marriage. If it is too cold you can bundle up and get out there and do what you must do if you want a better marriage, a great sex life and excellent communication.

7) Select the Type of Exercise

There are many different exercises that you are your husband or wife can do, but for the purpose of what we are trying to achieve here, some exercises are more suitable than others. The exercise you pick should be one that will allow you to talk to each other throughout the exercise. After you establish the habit of exercising together you can venture into other exercises. We have found from personal experience that running is one of the best exercises that will allow you talk to each other, because you can get close and there is little noise involved. If the weather is too hot, drees accordingly and face it squarely.

Based on our experience we highly recommend outdoor exercise because there are fewer interruptions and both of you will be able to talk to each other without interferences. But if you have a gym that is quite enough for you to exercise and talk you should go for it. Help is available and you can reach us through 90daysexercisechallenge@gmail.com.

How This Manual is Organized

This is a fairly easy to use manual. There are no prescribed activities for you are your husband or wife to do, but you have already been given an opportunity to select an activity or activities. The next big part of the manual is the daily discipline of meditating, exercising, and journaling. We felt that mental change drives physical change. This is why we include an inspirational quote for each day and a short meditation centered around the word of the day.

There is a check list of seven things that you need to keep an eye on five items on the list are done daily and the remaining two are done once a week. To get the most out of these 90 days you are required to follow the instructions in this manual to the best of your ability.

How to Use This Manual

Both husband and wife need their own copy of the manual because they will be required to journal during the 90 days period. At the end of each week both husband and wife will be required to compare the highlight of their journaling and adjust accordingly. Be ready for surprises about yourselves that are going to pop up for you will discover new things about yourselves. Here is the daily expected to do list;

1) Both of you are required to get up each day and read your why to each other.
2) Read the short daily devotional that is shared each day
3) Focus on the word of the day and let your conversation during the workout of that center around the word of the

day. Challenge each other on ways to incorporate the word of the day in your marriage.

4) Journaling is going to be a crucial part of this challenge.

5) Go out and exercise together. This is obvious right? But it is not going to come naturally, and you will have to push yourselves to make it happen.

6) Once a week both of you will sit down and evaluate how you are doing, what you have learned and adjustments that need to be made.

7) Once a week each one of you will take your weight and log it in the manual.

What Not to Do

The information in this manual is not meant for the couple down the street or for the Jones who you think need it more than you. If you are not exercising regular with your husband or wife this manual is for you and it should be used by both of you. It is imperative that both of you make this work. No matter how much you have fought in the past, now is the time for you to become a functional team for you need this to beat the odds.

This is a 90 days challenge and it is called a challenge because it is a challenge. You must get through the program for the 90 days if you want to get the reward. Do not allow the difficulties that will arise to prevent you from following through. Make sure that before you start the 90-day challenge you have blocked the time to do it, because you are required to finish it.

Monday: Forgiveness

*"There is no love without forgiveness, and
there is no forgiveness without love".*
Bryant H. McGill

We must start by talking about forgiveness, because it is a key component of any successful marriage. Without forgiveness past hurts will never heal and these wounds will become sceptic and can destroy your marriage. A story is told by Jesus of a servant who owed his master so much money to that he was unable to pay. Because of that the master ordered that the servant be thrown in jail until the debt was paid. The servant went on his knees and pleaded for mercy and for his debt to be forgiven. The master wrote of the debt and set the servant free. This servant was overjoyed, but his joy was short lived, when it occurred to him that one of his friends was owing him the equivalence of say $10. The servant who had been forgiven insisted that the other servant who was owing this small amount of money pay or be thrown into prison. The servant went on his knees and pledged for more time to be given to him, so he could pay back the money he was sowing. His cries fell on deaf ears, because the servant who had a debt of almost $1000,000 forgiven by their master insisted that the other servant be thrown in jail. When the servant was thrown in jail the other servants went and reported it to their master who had the unforgiving servant thrown in jail.

All of us including you and your husband or wife has and will make mistakes and the best thing to do for each other is to forgive. If you do not forgive you are imprisoning yourself and will eventually destroy your marriage and ultimately you. Draw some inspiration for the following Bible verse *"And whenever you stand praying, forgive, if you have anything against anyone, so that your Father also who is in heaven may forgive you your trespasses." Mark 11:25 (ESV)*

Daily To-Do List

1) Read your why to each other.
2) Read the short daily devotional and meditate
3) Take your weight and log it here: _____
4) Go out and exercise together
5) Focus on forgiveness and what that means to you and your relationship. Challenge each other during your exercise on ways to incorporate forgiveness in your marriage.
6) At the end of the day make a journal entry here on your observations and major takeaways.

_____

_____

_____

_____

_____

_____

_____

_____

_____

_____

_____

_____

_____

_____

_____

Day 2

Tuesday: Unforgiveness

*"Unforgiveness is like drinking poison yourself and
waiting for the other person to die."*
Marianne Williamson

Yesterday we saw the story of the unforgiving servant and the ending was not a good one. When people interact, they will step on each other's toes, therefore learning to forgive should be an integral part of every relationship. But you may be saying that, "I was hurt so badly that it makes no sense for me to forgive." We are telling you that it makes all the sense in the world for you to forgive because the price of unforgiveness is so high that you cannot afford to pay it, no matter how hard you try. In fact, unforgiveness is so costly that Jesus had the following response to peter when he has asked about people who wrong us multiple times.

*"Then Peter came up and said to him, "Lord, how often will my brother
sin against me, and I forgive him? As many as seven times?" Jesus said
to him, "I do not say to you seven times, but seventy times seven."
Mathew 18:21-22 (ESV)*

The response Jesus Christ gave to Peter must have surprised him. To forgive somebody 70 times 70 in a single day is equal to 490 times. This is a lot! You may take this figuratively or literally, but the bottom line is that you are required to forgive the same offended multiple times. In this case we are talking about your husband or wife who has caused you to be mad on multiple occasions. It is in your best interest to forgive, because the first person to benefit is you, then your relationship.

Daily to do list

1) Read your why to each other.
2) Read the short daily devotional and meditate
3) Go out and exercise together
4) Focus on unforgiveness and what that means to you and your relationship. Challenge each other during your exercise on ways to incorporate unforgiveness in your marriage.
5) At the end of the day make a journal entry here on your observations and major takeaways.

_____

_____

_____

_____

_____

_____

_____

_____

_____

_____

_____

_____

_____

_____

_____

Wednesday: Love

"Let us always meet each other with smile, for
the smile is the beginning of love."
Mother Teresa

Love is what brings two people together to get married in the first place and should be the glue that keeps them together. Love means many different things to different people, but you are going to be challenging to focus on this great love passage that Paul the apostle wrote the Corinthians

"If I speak in the tongues of men or of angels, but do not have love, I am only a resounding gong or a clanging cymbal. If I have the gift of prophecy and can fathom all mysteries and all knowledge, and if I have a faith that can move mountains, but do not have love, I am nothing. If I give all I possess to the poor and give over my body to hardship that I may boast, but do not have love, I gain nothing.

Love is patient, love is kind. It does not envy, it does not boast, it is not proud. It does not dishonor others, it is not self-seeking, it is not easily angered, it keeps no record of wrongs. Love does not delight in evil but rejoices with the truth. It always protects, always trusts, always hopes, always perseveres. Love never fails. But where there are prophecies, they will cease; where there are tongues, they will be stilled; where there is knowledge, it will pass away." 1 Corinthians 13 New International Version (NIV) Emphasis are mine.

This type of love Paul is describing here is agape love and it takes the Divine to love like this. You will have to encourage one another to let Divine love to flourish in your home.

Daily to do list

1) Read your why to each other.
2) Read the short daily devotional and meditate
3) Go out and exercise together
4) Focus on Divine love and what that means to you and your relationship. Challenge each other during your exercise on ways to incorporate Divine love in your marriage.
5) At the end of the day make a journal entry here on your observations and major takeaways.

_____

_____

_____

_____

_____

_____

_____

_____

_____

_____

_____

_____

_____

_____

_____

_____

Thursday: Sacrifice

"Human progress is neither automatic nor inevitable... Every step toward the goal of justice requires sacrifice, suffering, and struggle; the tireless exertions and passionate concern of dedicated individuals."
Martin Luther King, Jr.

Love and sacrifice go hand in hand, and it is not a bad thing to sacrifice for your love one. Husbands are challenged to lay down their lives for their wives as Christ did for the church. In other words, going the extra mile is recommended and encouraged. The quote that we are focusing on today is by Martin Luther King, Jr. Somebody who walked the talk and paid the ultimate sacrifice by laying down his life. One way to sacrifice in marriage is to learn your husband or wife's love language and speak it. This is extremely difficult because most of the time we want to do what we are comfort with and like to do. Take for example if your wife does not like you buying shoes for her or jewelry and clothes, you should not insist on doing that. The best thing to do is give her the money to go shop. This may sound easy enough, but many couples have stumbled because nobody is willing to sacrifice their preferences for the other. Have you heard of marriages break doing because of irreconcilable differences? What the husband and wife are saying is that we are not willing to sacrifice anything on behave of our marriage.

Both of you have been given the opportunity during this 9o day exercise challenge to sacrifice some of your comforts and habits for your marriage. Knowing is in doing and now is the opportunity to do just that.

Daily to do list

1) Read your why to each other.
2) Read the short daily devotional and meditate
3) Go out and exercise together
4) Focus on sacrifice and what that means to you and your relationship. Challenge each other during your exercise on ways to incorporate sacrifice in your marriage.
5) At the end of the day make a journal entry here on your observations and major takeaways.

_____

_____

_____

_____

_____

_____

_____

_____

_____

_____

_____

_____

_____

_____

_____

_____

_____

Day 5

Friday: Challenge

"No dream is too big. No challenge
is too great. Nothing we want for our
future is beyond our reach."
President Donald Trump

He is a summary of the troy story of Legson Kayira, who had a dream to come to the United States of America to further his education, but had not money, no contacts, and yet did the unthinkable. One early morning in the early 1960s he got up told his mother that he was going to walk to American and left his village in the then Nyasaland now present-day Malawi in East Africa and embarked on a journey that will take him halfway across the world on foot. It took him months and he had to overcome all sorts of obstacles, disease, hunger etc., but he made it to the United States of America and got a good education at Skagit Valley College in Washington State. Your marriage is worth over coming any challenge to ensure that it turns out right. Here is an opportunity for you to begin your own journey to a great marriage if you are not yet on it. Today you will be focusing on challenges, those you have face in the past and are facing right now. Our prayer for you is that you press on with this challenge and give it a technical knockout. The questions for you are, "What do you want for your marriage? What is your dream?" This is an opportunity to go behind that dream.

The quote above by the current United States of America President was made long before he ran to become the president of the greatest country on earth. Whatever you want for the future of your marriage is within your reach.

Daily to do list

1) Read your why to each other.
2) Read the short daily devotional and meditate
3) Go out and exercise together
4) Focus on sacrifice and what that means to you and your relationship. Challenge each other during your exercise on ways to incorporate sacrifice in your marriage.
5) At the end of the day make a journal entry here on your observations and major takeaways.

_____

_____

_____

_____

_____

_____

_____

_____

_____

_____

_____

_____

_____

_____

_____

Saturday: Courage

"Success is not final; failure is not fatal: it is the
courage to continue that counts."
Winston Churchill

Every great journey no matter how long it takes always depends on the first step. Some may wonder what has one step got to with a journey of a thousand miles. Well, the first step is the most important step, because every other step will never happen if the first step is not taken. In fact, there will be no journey to talk of if that first crucial step is no taking. How many dreams to you that have been killed because the dreamers lacked the courage to take the first step? They convinced themselves that either the dream was impossible to accomplish, or they were not having what it takes for them to accomplish it and so decided to do nothing. Failure only occurs when you stop trying or decide to give up. You are always one step away from a might breakthrough, that is why you have to keep moving. You are going to muster all the courage that you have and face this 90-day challenge. It must be done for you, your health, that of your partner and eventually your marriage.

It does not matter what stage you are in your marriage, there is room for improvement, and it is going to take courage to face all the obstacles that are standing on your way right now. Do not back down and never, never give up!

Daily to do list

1) Read your why to each other.
2) Read the short daily devotional and meditate
3) Go out and exercise together
4) Focus on forgiveness and what that means to you and your relationship. Challenge each other during your exercise on ways to incorporate forgiveness in your marriage.
5) At the end of the day make a journal entry here on your observations and major takeaways.

_____

_____

_____

_____

_____

_____

_____

_____

_____

_____

_____

_____

_____

_____

_____

_____

_____

Sunday: Determination

"I've always found that anything worth achieving will always have obstacles in the way and you've got to have that drive and determination to overcome those obstacles on route to whatever it is that you want to accomplish."
Chuck Norris

Congratulations! You have made it through a week. Your determination is paying off. The story is told about King David when he was a shepherd boy and his father sent him out to go give supplies to his brothers who were fighting against the philistines. When David arrived, the battle front he saw something that that made him to determine to do something about it in spite of the ridicule from his brothers. David saw giant from the enemy camp who was taunting and mocking the Israelites. Goliath the was so big that the entire Israeli army trembled when he stood up and challenged them to a send a man to come fight him. This went on for forty days and nobody had the courage to face him. Then David, the shepherd boy, shows up and decided to face the Goliath. David's brothers told him to go back and look after the sheep and accused him of trying to show off, but David was determined to bring down the giant, so he ignored his brothers, face Goliath and brought him down with a single and a single stone. We all have Goliaths in our lives that need to be defeated and all you need is determination. Do not listen to those who are mocking and making fun of you that you are trying to show off because you are trying to exercise together. Obstacles are expected, but you are not expected to let the obstacles stop you.

Daily to do list

1) Read your why to each other.
2) Read the short daily devotional and meditate
3) Take your weight and log it here_____
4) Go out and exercise together
5) Focus on determination and what that means to you and your relationship. Challenge each other during your exercise on ways to incorporate determination in your marriage.
6) At the end of the day make a journal entry here on your observations and major takeaways.
7) Both of you have to compare notes, evaluate your progress, and make adjustments accordingly.

_____

_____

_____

_____

_____

_____

_____

_____

_____

_____

_____

_____

_____

_____

_____

_____

Monday: Persistence

*"Nothing in this world can take the place of persistence. Talent will not:
nothing is more common than unsuccessful men with talent. Genius
will not; unrewarded genius is almost a proverb. Education will
not: the world is full of educated derelicts. Persistence
and determination alone are omnipotent."*
Calvin Coolidge

Have you been tempted to give up on your marriage? You are not alone. John was married to his high sweetheart immediately he graduated with his engineering degree and after three years they were having two children. Many people around them thought everything was going well, because each time John and Suzan were in the public, they were always smiling. But John was getting frustrated because all the efforts to make Suzan put off some weight were not paying off. The weight issue was not the only thing that was bothering John, Suzan who used to like having sex, out of sudden lost all interest and would rather spend time with their children. It got to the point where they were sleeping in separate rooms. Out of desperation John started contemplating the unthinkable. He wanted to walk away from the marriage and never comeback. Then he shared his struggles with a trusted friend who lovingly brought to John's attention that he had been working so hard on getting promoted at work that he had been there but not there. The quality of time that his wife, children, and marriage needed was not being given. The solution was for John to put first things first and all the other things will fall in place.

Daily to do list

1) Read your why to each other.
2) Read the short daily devotional and meditate
3) Go out and exercise together
4) Focus on persistency and what that means to you and your relationship. Challenge each other during your exercise on ways to incorporate persistency in your marriage.
5) At the end of the day make a journal entry here on your observations and major takeaways.

_____

_____

_____

_____

_____

_____

_____

_____

_____

_____

_____

_____

_____

_____

_____

_____

_____

Tuesday: Consistency

"I was always anti-marriage. I didn't understand monogamy. I couldn't figure out how that could last. And then I met Bryn, and I started to understand the beauty of constancy and history and change and going on the roller coaster with someone - of having a partner in life."
Maria Bello

Peter threw up his hands in desperation because he was having a hard time finishing the 5k that he had planned to over the weekend. Everything in him was telling him to stop running and out of sudden his body had become so heavy that it seemed as if he was wearing lead shoes. He was hyperventilating and at the point of passing out. To add salt to an injury, many participants, some way older than him and some younger than him all ran past him. Peter was in a sorry state because he had ignored a small yet profound principle, "the habits that you form will either make or break you." He was a little overweight for his age and out of shape because occasionally he went out for a walk but had never been consistent in exercising regularly. But had convinced himself that he could get up one day go out and run a 5k just like that! According, to him, as he told a colleague at work, it was just a 5K and he could handle it. Well, he was wrong! Because he blacked out and woke up in the emergency room at the hospital. The nurses explained to him how he had almost died.

It is not how much you do each time, but how long you are going to do it. That is why consistency must be built into your marriage and every other area of your life because it sets you to reap from the law of compound interest.

Daily to do list

1) Read your why to each other.
2) Read the short daily devotional and meditate
3) Go out and exercise together
4) Focus on consistency and what that means to you and your relationship. Challenge each other during your exercise on ways to incorporate consistency in your marriage.
5) At the end of the day make a journal entry here on your observations and major takeaways.

_____

_____

_____

_____

_____

_____

_____

_____

_____

_____

_____

_____

_____

_____

Day 10

Wednesday: Commitment

"Too many Christians have a commitment of convenience. They'll stay faithful as long as it's safe and doesn't involve risk, rejection, or criticism. Instead of standing alone in the face of challenge or temptation, they check to see which way their friends are going."
Charles Stanley

B ack in the day many people got married not because they had fallen in love. They started with commitment because their parents arranged for their marriages. We can spend all day arguing if this was a good idea or not and if these couples "truly enjoyed love". Fast forward to this day and age where there is so much talk about love, yet the divorce rate is going through the roof and the damage and destruction caused by divorce cannot be ignored. Many single parent homes, heartbreaks, disappoints and disillusionment with marriage are just some of the unwanted consequences of divorce. People who said they were so madly in love and will do everything for each other, become as cold as ice towards each other and to make matters worse, get on each other's nerves with the same intensity they "loved" each other. Some even kill because according to them, they love the other person so much that they want them dead. Love without commitment is fantasy and disaster waiting to happen. Ask all those who have been married for thirty plus years and are having a strong vibrant and blissful marriage what the secret of their success it and you will be supposed to hear that commitment ranks extremely high. It is OK to have feelings of love for your husband or wife, but these feelings are not enough. You need commitment of you want to go far. Now is an opportunity to commit to helping each other have, better health, save money, enjoy sex, and better communication.

Daily to do list

1) Read your why to each other.
2) Read the short daily devotional and meditate
3) Go out and exercise together
4) Focus on forgiveness and what that means to you and your relationship. Challenge each other during your exercise on ways to incorporate forgiveness in your marriage.
5) At the end of the day make a journal entry here on your observations and major takeaways.

_____

_____

_____

_____

_____

_____

_____

_____

_____

_____

_____

_____

_____

_____

_____

_____

Thursday: Dedication

*"It has not been easy to wake up every single
day at 6:30 in the morning to then head to the
gym and start a full day of work. But you have to
have that kind of dedication if you want to
achieve the goals you have set for yourself."*
Pablo Sandoval

Commitment produces dedication and you cannot have one without the other. You have to start with the commitment never to give up and to carry it to the end no matter what. When the commitment is made, then through dedication your commitment will be realized. We meet a lady the other day who has been exercising regularly for more than 40 years. My wife just came back from a funeral of one of our friend's mothers who had been married to his dad for 65 years. She died leaving behind her husband. To be married for 65 years is an excellent example of what commitment and dedication can produce. When you are dedicated you get up each day and do what you have committed to do. In this context we are talking about marriage and you have committed to loving your husband or wife and each day you have to show dedication to that committing of loving them through the highs and lows. You must keep going no matter what is thrown at you because you are dedicated. Both of you have committed to do this 90-day exercise challenge and it is going to take dedication for you to finish it. Commitment and dedication are not qualities that you pay lip service to. If you are committed and dedicated it will be obvious. This is one of those things that it is better to show than to talk about.

Show each other how committed and dedicated you are to a strong and vibrant marriage by completing this challenge.

Daily to do list

1) Read your why to each other.
2) Read the short daily devotional and meditate
3) Go out and exercise together
4) Focus on forgiveness and what that means to you and your relationship. Challenge each other during your exercise on ways to incorporate forgiveness in your marriage.
5) At the end of the day make a journal entry here on your observations and major takeaways.

_____

_____

_____

_____

_____

_____

_____

_____

_____

_____

_____

_____

_____

_____

_____

_____

Friday: Faithfulness

*"Marriage has a unique place because it speaks of an absolute
faithfulness, a covenant between radically different persons, male
and female; and so, it echoes the absolute covenant of God with his
chosen, a covenant between radically different partners."*
Rowan Williams

Jake was deployed to the south east theater during the second
world war to fight against the Japanese. Two weeks before his
deployment he and his high school sweetheart got married. On the
night before Jake was deployed, he and Linda promised each other
that no matter what happens they will love each other faithfully until
death parts them. There were two main concerns on their minds, the
possibility of Jake being killed or sustaining serious injurious at war.
The next day they tearfully said goodbye to each other as Jake gave
her the last hug and kiss. After about a month Linda received a letter
from Jake informing her of the situation he was in and how much he
loved her. That was going to be the last letter she will receive from
him. Linda waited and waited and got no news whatsoever from
her beloved husband and the months of waiting turned into years
as the war dragged on. She was worried, lonely and each day she
feared for the worst. In fact, a few of her friend's husbands had been
killed already and the folder flag had been delivered to them. In the
fourth year after her husband's deployment she ran into one of her
former high school mates who started making advances towards her
and trying to take her out on a date. He insisted that it was unfair
for Jake to be gone for so long without any communication and
that since they were not having any children, she should start her a

new life with him. Linda refused and told him never to contact her again. She had given a promise to Jake and will wait no matter what. Her faithfulness paid off because a few months after the end of the war Jake knocked at the door and explained to her why she had not received any letters from him.

Daily to do list

1) Read your why to each other.
2) Read the short daily devotional and meditate
3) Go out and exercise together
4) Focus on faithfulness
5) and what that means to you and your relationship. Challenge each other during your exercise on ways to incorporate faithfulness in your marriage.
6) At the end of the day make a journal entry here on your observations and major takeaways.

_____

_____

_____

_____

_____

_____

_____

_____

_____

_____

_____

_____

_____

Saturday: Surrender

"Romantic love can be terrifying. We experience another human being as enormously important to us. So, there is surrender – not a surrender to the other person so much as to our feeling for the other person. What is the obstacle? The possibility of loss."
Nathaniel Branden

You might have grown up hearing that you should never surrender. There is a place for never surrendering and you should never surrender in the face of opposition, abuse, neglect, or injustice. Anything that threatens your life or the wellbeing of your family, friends or other people should be opposed by all and at all times. But this is not the type of surrounding we are talking about here. We are referring to your willing and out of your free violation surrendering yourself to another person. This does not mean you become a servant or take second place. It means that you surrender your right to payback, your right to be right or win the argument. For you to be successful on this 90-day challenge both of you will have to do some surrendering. It may be as easy as giving up your preference of exercising in the night, or swimming over running.

Both of you should identify all the excuses and perceived obstacles that have been preventing you from exercising and surrender them. Now is the time to give them up so that you can embark on this life changing journey that has the potential of taking your marriage to the next level. In this contest sundering is a good thing to do and it is not an indication that you have failed. Only the strong know when to surrender and we know you are strong and will do anything to safeguard your marriage. So, do it by surrendering!

Daily to do list

1) Read your why to each other.
2) Read the short daily devotional and meditate
3) Go out and exercise together
4) Focus on surrender and what that means to you and your relationship. Challenge each other during your exercise on ways to incorporate surrender in your marriage.
5) At the end of the day make a journal entry here on your observations and major takeaways.

_____

_____

_____

_____

_____

_____

_____

_____

_____

_____

_____

_____

_____

_____

_____

Sunday: Surrender

"We shall defend our island, whatever the cost may be, we shall fight on the beaches, we shall fight on the landing grounds, we shall fight in the fields and in the streets, we shall fight in the hills; we shall never surrender."
Winston Churchill

In 1940 Hitler was at the height of his conquest, because it had taken him just six weeks to defeat the French army and occupy France. His next target was Great Britain and Hitler was bent on occupying the Island because it was the last frontier in Western Europe that the Germans had not occupied. The Germans were so confident of the superiority of their air force the Luftwaffe, the head Hermann Goering thought the British Royal Air Force (RAF) was going to be destroyed in just four days. Hitler had been hoping that the British will just surrender after the humiliating defeat of the French army but when this did not happen, he launched Operation Sea Lion, with the intent of defeating and occupying Great Britain. It was vital for Operation Sea Lion to succeed because Hitler did not want Britain to be used as a base to fight the German, should the United States of America enter the war.

This is the backdrop of why Winston Churchill the British Prime Minster at that time railed his people with this famous quote about fighting and never surrendering. You too should not surrender to anything that will try to come against, your health, finance and marriage. Fight!

Daily to do list

1) Read your why to each other.
2) Read the short daily devotional and meditate
3) Take your weight and log it here: _____
4) Go out and exercise together
5) Focus on surrender and what that means to you and your relationship. Challenge each other during your exercise on ways to incorporate surrender in your marriage.
6) At the end of the day make a journal entry here on your observations and major takeaways.
7) Both of you have to compare notes, evaluate your progress, and make adjustments accordingly.

_____

_____

_____

_____

_____

_____

_____

_____

_____

_____

_____

_____

_____

_____

Day 15

Monday: Conquer

"When you start in life, if you find you are wrongly placed, don't hesitate to change, but don't change because troubles come up and difficulties arise. You must meet and overcome and conquer them. And in meeting and overcoming and conquering them, you will make yourself stronger for the future."
Charles M. Schwab

The only way you conquer is by being courageous fighting and not surrendering to an enemy no matter what or who the enemy is. If there are no obstacles on your path there will be nothing to to overcome. If there is no war declared against you there will be no battle to fight and no enemy to defeat and conquer. Therefore, do not panic if your marriage is facing a lot of internal and external opposition. It was not matter what the source of the problem is, what matter is that you must fight and conquer all. We are hoping that this journey will equip you to fight and defeat any enemy that may be position against your health, and marriage. There is no substitute to victory, for the only alternative is defeat which will cost you your health, life and eventually marriage. How can you be married when you are dead? The answer is obvious. You cannot be dead and married at the same time. To avoid this from happening, it is crucial that you take care of your health and you and your husband or wife can help each other to do that. If you can do all to conquer whatever obstacles you are facing right now and build the habit of exercising together as couple you are securing a brighter future for your finances, health, and marriage. Therefore, what you do today will determine what the future will hold for you. We are hoping that you will do the right thing by continuing to exercise with your husband or wife.

Daily to do list

1) Read your why to each other.
2) Read the short daily devotional and meditate
3) Go out and exercise together
4) Focus on forgiveness and what that means to you and your relationship. Challenge each other during your exercise on ways to incorporate forgiveness in your marriage.
5) At the end of the day make a journal entry here on your observations and major takeaways.

_____

_____

_____

_____

_____

_____

_____

_____

_____

_____

_____

_____

_____

_____

Day 16

Tuesday: Defeat

"The most beautiful people we have known are those who have known defeat, known suffering, known struggle, known loss, and have found their way out of those depths."
Elisabeth Kubler-Ross

Here is a snapshot in the life of Abraham Lincoln the Sixteenth president of the United States of America, a man who suffered many defeats, yet eventually occupied the greatest office on the land; the presidency of the United States of America.

In 1832 he lost his job and was defeated in a run for the state legislature. The next year 1833 his business failed, in 1935 his sweetheart died, and he had a nervous breakdown in 1836. Somehow, he got elected into the Illinois House of Assemble but run 1838 to be the Speaker of the house and was defeated. The next big move for him was to go to the United States Congress in 1843, again he was defeated during the nomination for congress. After five years in 1848 he tried again to run for congress and was defeated during the nomination a second time. A year later in 1848 he tried to become a land officer but was rejected. Five years later in 1854 he rand for the United States of America senate and was defeated. Two years later in 1856 he was defeated for the nomination for vice president of the United States of America. In 1858 he suffered another defeat as he ran for the US senate. After about 11 defeats or call them setbacks over a period of 28 years Abraham Lincoln triumphed and was elected the sixteenth president of the United States of America in 1860. [1]

You and your husband or wife might have been through many defeats, but have persevered, be encouraged this challenge may just be what you need for a turnaround. This is your opportunity to triumph over any odds that may be against you and your marriage. Do not allow any past defeats no matter how many or devastating they were to stop you. Both of you have what it takes to win and win big!

Daily to do list

1) Read your why to each other.
2) Read the short daily devotional and meditate
3) Go out and exercise together
4) Focus on defeat and what that means to you and your relationship. Challenge each other during your exercise on ways to incorporate defeat in your marriage.
5) At the end of the day make a journal entry here on your observations and major takeaways.

_____

_____

_____

_____

_____

_____

_____

_____

_____

_____

---

[1] *http://www.abrahamlincolnonline.org/lincoln/education/failures.htm*

Day 17

Wednesday: Enemy

"Listen! Clam up your mouth and be silent like an oyster shell, for that tongue of yours is the enemy of the soul, my friend. When the lips are silent, the heart has a hundred tongues."
Rumi

It is human nature to point to others our circumstances and external environment as the source of our problems. Most people will blame everybody, anything, and everything, but seldomly point any finger at them. They forget that each time you point one finger at somebody else four fingers are pointing back at you. There may be an external enemy, but the internal enemy is the deadliest. Therefore, it is incumbent on you to accept that there is an internal enemy, then identify it and deal with it accordingly. Failure to do so, implies that you are going to be trapped for life and it will cause you, your health and eventually marriage. Now is the time to stop looking on the outside and focus on the inside. What are some of the negative self-limiting believes you hold about yourself? What are some of the things you have told yourself are impossible to be accomplished? You cannot fight and defeat an enemy you do not know. Do you know that you are your greatest enemy? How do you expect people to believe you when you do not believe yourself? How will your marriage flourish you believe that the marriage if not worth working and fighting for? Who are you expecting to stand and defend your marriage? If you treat your marriage as a piece of junk how do you expect it to be honored by others who are having nothing at stake or anything to lose if your marriage fails. Now is the time to accept that your greatest enemy is you and it is you and you alone that has to confront this internal enemy and defeat it. The good thing is that you can do and will do it successfully if you take responsibility.

Daily to do list

1) Read your why to each other.
2) Read the short daily devotional and meditate
3) Go out and exercise together
4) Focus on forgiveness and what that means to you and your relationship. Challenge each other during your exercise on ways to incorporate forgiveness in your marriage.
5) At the end of the day make a journal entry here on your observations and major takeaways.

_____

_____

_____

_____

_____

_____

_____

_____

_____

_____

_____

_____

_____

_____

_____

_____

Thursday: Time

*"Your time is limited, so don't waste it living someone else's life.
Don't be trapped by dogma – which is living with the results of
other people's thinking. Don't let the noise of others' opinions
drown out your own inner voice. And most important,
have the courage to follow your heart and intuition."*
Steve Jobs

You do not have all the time in the world and should treat each day as your last day. As uncomfortable as this may sound, the truth is that your life is the sum of each day. Therefore, do all to make each day count. Yesterday is gone and tomorrow is not guaranteed; now is all you have and should not waste it. Many marriages are stagnant because both the husband and wife are waiting for the right conditions and the perfect day to start truly taking care of the marriage. Some are waiting to make more money, some for a promotion and advancement; others are waiting for their children to grow and leave the house before they will rekindle their love and grow it. Nobody has promised you that you are going to live to a certain age and now is the time to start maximizing every day that is given to both of you. We talked about forgiveness and the need to let go of the past already and you are highly encouraged to forgive each and not allow your past to rob you of your day and eventually your tomorrow. Here are some wise words spoken by King David under the inspiration of the Holy Spirit as recorded in the book of Psalms

*"Teach us to number our days, that we
may gain a heart of wisdom."*
Psalm 90:12"

Have you numbered your days? Do you number your days daily?
Are you aware of the fact that your days are indeed number and each
passing day you are getting closer to your grave? If today was going
to be your last day how will you like to be remembered?

Daily to do list

1) Read your why to each other.
2) Read the short daily devotional and meditate
3) Go out and exercise together
4) Focus on time and what that means to you and your
   relationship. Challenge each other during your exercise on
   ways to incorporate time in your marriage.
5) At the end of the day make a journal entry here on your
   observations and major takeaways.

_____

_____

_____

_____

_____

_____

_____

_____

_____

_____

_____

Friday: Purpose

"Being busy does not always mean real work. The object of all work is production or accomplishment and to either of these ends there must be forethought, system, planning, intelligence, and honest purpose, as well as perspiration. Seeming to do is not doing."
Thomas A. Edison

Why did you get marry to the person you are married to? What is it that both of you want to accomplish? What is keeping both of you married? These a obvious questions and you may be wondering why these questions should be asked in the first place. You are right in thinking like that, for the assumption is that all married couples must have figured out the answers to these questions. Unfortunately, the reality is that most have not, and the evidence is manifested through the high divorce rate we are experiencing. If there is no purpose to getting married, then there is no need to get married in the first place. After you get married if there is no purpose staying married to any particular individual the obvious action is to divorce and go your separate ways. If any married husband and wife do not know what is keeping them together, they will not know how to maintain nourish and grow the intimacy in their marriage and sooner or later will drift apart as many marriages are doing right now.

By now you are familiar with you why of embarking on this 90-day exercise challenge and have started experiencing the power of a powerful why. Your marriage needs a strong why that will drive the purpose of the two of you staying together married. When you establish your why and purpose no matter what is thrown at you, you will be unstoppable.

Daily to do list

1) Read your why to each other.
2) Read the short daily devotional and meditate
3) Go out and exercise together
4) Focus on purpose and what that means to you and your relationship. Challenge each other during your exercise on ways to incorporate purpose in your marriage.
5) At the end of the day make a journal entry here on your observations and major takeaways.

_____

_____

_____

_____

_____

_____

_____

_____

_____

_____

_____

_____

_____

_____

_____

_____

_____

Day 20

Saturday: Sowing

"Did I offer peace today? Did I bring a smile to someone's face? Did I say words of healing? Did I let go of my anger and resentment? Did I forgive? Did I love? These are the real questions. I must trust that the little bit of love that I sow now will bear many fruits, here in this world and the life to come."
Henri Nouwen

Ambe is one of those employees that everybody at work likes to ask out for lunch and when he has function in his house people from all works of life show up. There is something about him that seems to draw people to him and many of his friends have asked him how he does it. Ambe who migrated from the North Western region of Cameron in West Africa to the United States of America was raised in a Christian home. He recalls the extensive lessons his Grandma thought him while he was a child. Each morning Ambe was expected to go to the stream and fetch, but he did not like it and grumbled a lot. Then one cold and raining morning Ambe went to the stream with their priced calabash to fech some water, got in a serious argument with one of the other children and they got in a fight while walking back home. Ambe placed the calabash on the ground and as he was wrestling with the other boy, both of them fell on the calabash and broke it. Ambe came him in tears and his father gave him a whooping of his life. It was so sore from the beatings he received that he missed school for two days. During those two days and Ambe's grandmother was nursing his wounds she told in about the importance of having the right attitude and sowing the right seeds, both in our lives and the lives of others, because what you sow is what you get. This lesson hit home for him because in his village of substance farmers, he witnessed firsthand the practical application of this lesson. Ambe resolved to sow good seeds all the time, be being kind, polite, helpful, caring and loving to all people he meets.

Daily to do list

1) Read your why to each other.
2) Read the short daily devotional and meditate
3) Go out and exercise together
4) Focus on sowing and what that means to you and your relationship. Challenge each other during your exercise on ways to sowing forgiveness in your marriage.
5) At the end of the day make a journal entry here on your observations and major takeaways.

_____

_____

_____

_____

_____

_____

_____

_____

_____

_____

_____

_____

_____

_____

Day 21

Sunday: Reap

"If we don't plant the right things, we will reap the wrong things. It goes without saying. And you don't have to be, you know, a brilliant biochemist and you don't have to have an IQ of 150. Just common sense tells you to be kind, ninny, fool."
Be kind. Maya Angelou

When you get up each day, it is an opportunity to sow seeds and allow time to work for you and not against you. Size every opportunity that is given to you to plant seeds that will bring the type of fruit that you will like to eat. Nobody wants, anger, strive, hatred, jealousy, bitterness, resentment, envy, murder etc., But why do you sow these things in your marriage and expect to reap, peace, joy, happiness, faithfulness, fulfillment, contentment etc.? Have you not heard the following?

"Do not be deceived: God cannot be mocked.
A man reaps what he sows."
Galatians 6:7

This Bible verse is emphatically clear that you cannot plant apples and expect to harvest oranges. You must sow apples to reap apples and anything else you do is living in self-deceit. If your marriage is as important as you say it is, now is the time to show by your actions that you mean what you say. Congratulations! You have reached the 21-day mark and the habit of exercising as a couple is being strengthen and hopefully it will take hold of both of you and you will reap good health, excellent communication and great sex. Your marriage is going to grow in intimacy and your love for each other with be deepen as well. You will reap what you sow, therefore sow wisely.

Daily to do list

1) Read your why to each other.
2) Read the short daily devotional and meditate
3) Take your weight and log it here_____
4) Go out and exercise together
5) Focus on reap and what that means to you and your relationship. Challenge each other during your exercise on ways to incorporate reaping in your marriage.
6) At the end of the day make a journal entry here on your observations and major takeaways.
7) Both of you have to compare notes, evaluate your progress and make adjustments accordingly.

_____

_____

_____

_____

_____

_____

_____

_____

_____

_____

_____

_____

_____

Day 22

Monday: Hope

"Our uniqueness, our individuality, and our life experience molds us into fascinating beings. I hope we can embrace that. I pray we may all challenge ourselves to delve into the deepest resources of our hearts to cultivate an atmosphere of understanding, acceptance, tolerance, and compassion. We are all in this life together."
Linda Thompson

When we have a strong why and a life of purpose hope is going to be our constant companion because we have something to look forward to in the future. The intensity with which today is engaged is fueled by the possibilities that the future holds for us. We are not afraid to put in our all to make today great because we know the seeds that are being sowed today will bring us a bountiful harvest tomorrow. We believe enough in a better future to not squander today. Amina has only one son and decided to invest all she had to educate him. But most of her neighbors and other inhabitants of her village laughed at her for wasting her resources in educating her son. Many told her nothing good will come out of it, and money will serve her better if she saved it and got a wife for his son instead. Amina who was not educated believed that education was going to be the game changer for her and her son. While others were spending their money on the latest goods in the market, she was investing in the education of her son. All she hung on was the endless possibilities that education will open for her and her son. At the end of the year during the festivities where everybody bought new clothes, not let that bother her, because her priorities were different. Finally, her son graduated from the All Saints Technical Institute with a degree in civil engineering and all her investment and hard work paid off. It did not take long for her son to build a new house in the village for her. She became the talk of the village because she was having the only corrugated iron roof meanwhile the rest of the houses in the village were mud huts with thatch roofs. There is nothing as powerful as living with hope for the future. You must continue to be hopeful about the future of your marriage no matter what is going on now.

Daily to do list

1) Read your why to each other.
2) Read the short daily devotional and meditate
3) Go out and exercise together
4) Focus on hope and what that means to you and your relationship. Challenge each other during your exercise on ways to incorporate hope in your marriage.
5) At the end of the day make a journal entry here on your observations and major takeaways.

_____

_____

_____

_____

_____

_____

_____

_____

_____

_____

_____

Tuesday: Peace

"People respond in accordance to how you relate to them. If you approach them on the basis of violence, that's how they'll react. But if you say, 'We want peace, we want stability,' we can then do a lot of things that will contribute towards the progress of our society."
Nelson Mandela

There is so much yearning for peace, many books have been written and songs sang calling on all of us to just get along. But the reality is different from what all of desire, because we allow other things to get into the way. Fear is one of the greatest enemies of peace. When we allow fear to inform our decisions, we end up taking actions that are contrary to bring peace in our lives and those around us. As a couple your desire should be to have peace in your home and marriage. Before we fight for world peace, let us start with peace at home. For if all homes were peaceful the world will be more peaceful. Unfortunately, the reality is that many marriages are war zones because most couples are fighting over control, money, and dominance. Cultivating an atmosphere of peace at home should be your number one priority because without peace and tranquility in your home other aspects of your lives will surfer. Take the case of Pete who never comes home after work on time but stops at the bar to drink away his misery. Pete will drink and drink to the brink of passing out and drag himself home after everybody was already in bed. His children never get to see him and his wife who sleeps in a separate room wonders how long their marriage was going to last. Their troubles a had started after Pete lost his first job and took to drinking to ease his pain. Initially he said, he was going to stop because each time he drank and came home drunk he will be verbally abusive to his wife. Eventually he found a new job, buy alcohol had taken over his life and enslaved him to the point where he had to drink peace day. Their marriage took a beating and peace left their home. Now they are considering divorce and the only thing that is keeping them together are their children.

Daily to do list

1) Read your why to each other.
2) Read the short daily devotional and meditate
3) Go out and exercise together
4) Focus on peace and what that means to you and your relationship. Challenge each other during your exercise on ways to incorporate peace in your marriage.
5) At the end of the day make a journal entry here on your observations and major takeaways.

———————————————————————————

———————————————————————————

———————————————————————————

———————————————————————————

———————————————————————————

———————————————————————————

———————————————————————————

———————————————————————————

———————————————————————————

———————————————————————————

———————————————————————————

———————————————————————————

———————————————————————————

Wednesday: Faith

*"Faith is taking the first step even when
you don't see the whole staircase."*
Martin Luther King, Jr.

No word has been distorted caricatured, misused, and misunderstood as the word faith. It is unfortunate that some have gone to the extent of thinking that anything to do with faith lacks intellectual prowess, thoughtfulness, commonsense, facts and evidence. The truth is far from this. Faith has nothing to do with feelings, emotions, or wishful thinking, because there is nothing as faith in faith itself. Faith is always based on something and your faith is only as good as the object of your faith. Those who define faith as a leap in the dark or jumping over a chasm without any knowledge are misguided. If you take a look at what Martin Luther King Jr. is saying, your realize that before you take the first step on the staircase there must be a staircase to start with, even though you do not see the entire staircase you know from experience that staircases have a beginning and an end. Your past interaction with normal staircases has informed you that they always lead somewhere. Armed with all this knowledge and experience you can take that first steep with confidence because you know it will deliver. Here is one of the most powerful and succinct definitions of faith;

*"Now faith is confidence in what we hope for and
assurance about what we do not see."*
Hebrews 11:1 NIV

There is confidence involved and we know if something is not trustworthy, reliable, and dependable we cannot have confidence in. When you have an assurance for anything, it is depending on who is giving you the assurance and not how you feel. We are hoping that you will build a strong marriage that both of you can have faith in. Above all you should have faith in God as well and He will lead and guide you in your marriage.

Daily to do list

1) Read your why to each other.
2) Read the short daily devotional and meditate
3) Go out and exercise together
4) Focus on faith and what that means to you and your relationship. Challenge each other during your exercise on ways to incorporate faith in your marriage.
5) At the end of the day make a journal entry here on your observations and major takeaways.

_____

_____

_____

_____

_____

_____

_____

_____

_____

_____

_____

_____

Thursday: Perseverance

"I think you make the best with what you've got, you know? Sometimes you have very little. And you just always try to rise to higher ground, because you're going to suffer one way or the other, so you just hope that you have strength and perseverance and good friends and faith, some kind of faith, to endure and move on to greener pastures."
Pierce Brosnan

The ability to persevere is going to set your marriage apart from many other marriages. You do not talk about preference you demonstrate it. Talk is cheap but those who preserve walk the talk no matter how long or difficult it takes for them to do what they said they were going to do. When you meet your wife or husband you made some promises that might have sounded outlandish, but you did anyway and as the years have gone by you wish you had not made them. Part of the reason is that going is getting tough and the logical conclusion for you is to backout. After all there were just words that were altered, and your partner will understand if you do not follow through. You have to keep your word and perseverance is how you do it. Remind yourself that you made the promise and you must keep it. There is no substitute to perseverance when it comes to building a solid marriage. Many couples give up to soon because they have not understood the power of perseverance. Nobody said marriage was going to be a piece of cake and devoid of any difficulties and challenges. If your marriage is like that please, we will like you to share with the rest of us how you did it. Those who preserve know that the marriage is tough, yet they toughen up and keep going no matter what is thrown at them. They keep their eyes on the price and do not let their circumstances dictate what they do. It is impossible to stop a couple that have allowed perseverance to talk permeance in their marriage. While marriages are falling apart around them, they wax stronger and stronger with each passing day, because there is no room for failure in their marriage. In short, their marriage is divorce-proof and will last for a long time.

Daily to do list

1) Read your why to each other.
2) Read the short daily devotional and meditate
3) Go out and exercise together
4) Focus on perseverance and what that means to you and your relationship. Challenge each other during your exercise on ways to incorporate perseverance in your marriage.
5) At the end of the day make a journal entry here on your observations and major takeaways.

_____

_____

_____

_____

_____

_____

_____

_____

_____

_____

_____

_____

_____

Friday: Romance

"Husbands and wives, first be faithful to each other. Second, keep the romance going all of your life by courting each other every day."
Zig Ziglar

While they were in courtship Jim unfailing brought her flowers, gifts and each Friday evening they had a date night. During their dates they will just sit down and talk to each other for hours o end and it was so exciting. At times they repeated the same stories, but it was not boring to listen to them. When Jim got up each morning before he left the house he will call and check to see how she sleep because they were not yet married and were living in different parts of the city. In their minds Jim and Annette thought when they eventually get married and are living under the same roof and sharing the same bed, their romance will intensify, because they will be able to stay up all night especially over the weekends and talk as long as they want. Jim usually drove for almost an hour to come pick her up for their date night, when they get marry this one hour of commute time will be invested in the relationship.

Jim and Annette did not have to wait for a lifetime to test their hypothesis, because after one year of bliss, they got married. Their honeymoon location was carefully chosen to ensure that they started their marriage with a blast. Immediately the guests left the wedding reception, they boarded a plane and headed to the Caribbean where they had so much fun that they felt like remining therefore ever. They kept telling each other that marriage is so good and they is no excuse why any couple should divorce. Immediately they came back from the honey money the issues started, because Jim had to put in extra hours at work to cover part of the cost of the weeding and Anette started working to chip in to cover the other bills. Not too long both of them will return home tired and worn out and all they wanted to do was go to bed and rest. This continued to a while and once in a while they will promise to get back to "normalcy", but it never happened and right now Jim and Annette are contemplating the unthinkable. Divorce!

Daily to do list

1) Read your why to each other.
2) Read the short daily devotional and meditate
3) Go out and exercise together
4) Focus on romance and what that means to you and your relationship. Challenge each other during your exercise on ways to incorporate romance in your marriage.
5) At the end of the day make a journal entry here on your observations and major takeaways.

Day 27

Saturday: Intimacy

"In my mind, marriage is a spiritual partnership and union in which we willingly give and receive love, create and share intimacy, and open ourselves to be available and accessible to another human being in order to heal, learn and grow."
Iyanla Vanzant

The key word here is willingly. It is impossible to have intimacy without the willingness to receive and give love, affection, and romance. Like other great things that build marriages, intimacy will not just happen. Both of you will have to put in some hard work and effort to grow in intimacy. There are so many things that are acting against your marriage and doing all within their power to keep you apart. The closer a couple gets that more difficult it is for their marriage to fall apart and the more the potential for forgiveness, healing, restoration, and growth. We are hoping that you are going to grow closer to each other during this 90-day challenge. The good news is that when you exercise your release the love hormone oxytocin which helps the two of you to bond and get closer. This is why are strongly recommend that you are you wife or husband should exercise together and consistently during these 90 days and hopeful by the end of the 90-day challenge you will form that habit that will take you throughout life. You cannot go wrong exercising together. Unfortunately, intimacy is under serve attack because of our modern lifestyle.

Take the case of Andrew and Maria who thought their relationship was invincible before they get married, but when they started having children and Andrew took a regional sales position that demand frequent travelling, their intimacy went south. Initially they tried to leverage technology by having facetime, chatting and frequent calls, but as time went on things just slowly deteriorated to the point where when Andrew comes home, he feels as if he is a stranger in his own house.

Daily to do list

1) Read your why to each other.
2) Read the short daily devotional and meditate
3) Go out and exercise together
4) Focus on intimacy and what that means to you and your relationship. Challenge each other during your exercise on ways to incorporate intimacy in your marriage.
5) At the end of the day make a journal entry here on your observations and major takeaways.

_____

_____

_____

_____

_____

_____

_____

_____

_____

_____

_____

_____

Sunday: Sex

*"There is no age limit on the enjoyment of
sex. It keeps getting better."*
Florence Henderson

Why does the subject of sex make so many people uncomfortable? "Normal" people do not talk about what happens in the bedroom under the sheets. We know that married people have sex, yet it is not a topic that is discussed freely. Sex is one of the indicators of health of a marriage. You can quickly access the quality of any marriage by the quality of the sex both the husband and wife are having. On the scale of 1 to 10 how do you rate your sex life. One being cold and 10 very hot. Where do you fall on this scale? What are some of the things that have made your sex life cold? When Zack got married to Suzi they could not keep their hands off each other or keep their clothes on when they were at home. Then the first child came in followed by the second and the third. In short, their lives became hectic with the demands of work, child rearing and they unconsciously place sex on the back burner. Because most of the times there was no time for it and when time was available, they were too tired to have sex. Unknowing to them their intimacy was reducing as well. Occasionally they will make up and promise to do more, but other demands on their time choked sex out. After the last child left for college, Zac and Suzi tried hard to rekindle the sex they had neglected for many years and it did not workout. At the heart of their frustration was resentment, hurt and bitterness that had remained unattended to over the years. They had waited for too long and grown apart from each other, what had been keeping together was their children and now that the children were all gone, they could no longer stay together. This is how this couple separated after 34 years of marriage.

Daily to do list

1) Read your why to each other.
2) Read the short daily devotional and meditate
3) Take your weight and log it here: _____
4) Go out and exercise together
5) Focus on sex and what that means to you and your relationship. Challenge each other during your exercise on ways to incorporate sex in your marriage.
6) At the end of the day make a journal entry here on your observations and major takeaways.
7) Both of you have to compare notes, evaluate your progress, and make adjustments accordingly.

_____

_____

_____

_____

_____

_____

_____

_____

_____

_____

_____

_____

_____

Monday: Trust

"I believe that a trusting attitude and a patient attitude go hand in hand. You see, when you let go and learn to trust God, it releases joy in your life. And when you trust God, you're able to be more patient. Patience is not just about waiting for something... it's about how you wait, or your attitude while waiting."
Joyce Meyer

Without trust it is impossible to build a solid and lasting marriage. Both husband and wife have to be trustworthy for this to happen. Do you trust each other? To be trustworthy means that you are reliable and dependable. The only way you can do this is being keeping your word and when you make promises you follow through. Matt meet Angelica a wedding reception for one of his friends and it was love at first sight. After three months they were married. On the first night of their honeymoon Matt told Angelica that trust was something that was dear to him and for their marriage to last, they must incorporate it in the marriage from day one. He went on to explain to her that he had a secret that he has been carrying for years that nobody knows, but now that they are married, she has to be know because a lot depends on it. Before now Anglica knew that Matt was a business owner and was doing very well, but she did not know that there was more to it than the eyes could see. Now Matt was about to lay everything on the line for their marriage. He opened one of the suitcases took out and alabaster box and told Angelica that the secrete for his business success was stored in the box and it should never be opened no matter what happens. Because the day the box is opened, he was going to go broke. Angelica assured

Matt that he could trust her, for she will never open the alabaster box. After their honeymoon Matt and Angelica went home and not too long hard one of those arguments that couples have and it tempers flared and Angelica ran into the room, grabbed the alabaster box, and threaten to open it. Matt fall on his knees pleaded and cried that she should not open it, Anglica was so angry that she opened the box.

Daily to do list

1) Read your why to each other.
2) Read the short daily devotional and meditate
3) Go out and exercise together
4) Focus on trust and what that means to you and your relationship. Challenge each other during your exercise on ways to incorporate trust in your marriage.
5) At the end of the day make a journal entry here on your observations and major takeaways.

_____

_____

_____

_____

_____

_____

_____

_____

_____

_____

_____

_____

Tuesday: Reliability

"Facts from paper are not the same as facts from people. The reliability of the people giving you the facts is as important as the facts themselves."
Harold S. Geneen

Our first car was a 1992 Toyota corolla and had a lot of mechanical problems. One of the most annoying ones that developed a few months after the car was bought had to do with the starter. The first time that problem occurred, was at a traffic light where I had stopped because the light was red. After the light changed to green, the engine of the car shot off and I frantically tried to start to car but was unsuccessful. To make matters worse, the summer heat was making the temperature in the car to rise at an alarming rate. After what appeared to be ages I tried to start the car again and the engine came alive. I drove home, but being students at that time, we could not see a mechanic to check the car to find out what had caused it to stop suddenly and why it started after a while. Not too long after that, we drove the car to visit a friend and when our visit was over we got into the car and tried to start it, but the car would not start. We kept trying and finally succeeded to start the car. After encountering this problem on many different occasions, it occurred to us that it was miss and hit, since at times the car will start and other times it will not, and we will have to wait for and at times pour water on some parts of the engine to cool it, because we had figured out that it helps the car to start. In short, our car was unreliable, and we could not count on it to start unfailingly each we wanted it to. We finally scraped some money together for the car to be repaired. When the repair was done we never had that problem again. The car became reliable and will start each time we turn the ignition on.

Are you reliable? Can your mate depend on you to be there for them and for you to do what you have promised them you are going to do?

Daily to do list

1) Read your why to each other.
2) Read the short daily devotional and meditate
3) Go out and exercise together
4) Focus on reliability and what that means to you and your relationship. Challenge each other during your exercise on ways to incorporate reliability in your marriage.
5) At the end of the day make a journal entry here on your observations and major takeaways.

_____

_____

_____

_____

_____

_____

_____

_____

_____

_____

_____

_____

_____

Wednesday: Promise

"In the 1960s, if you introduced a new product to America, 90% of the people who viewed it for the first time believed in the corporate promise. Then 40 years later if you performed the same exercise, less than 10% of the public believed it was true. The fracturing of trust is based on the fact that the consumer has been let down."
Howard Schultz

Of what use is a promise that is not kept? The hope that a promise offers is only as good as the ability of the person who offered the promise to keep it. Are a man or woman of your word? Can you husband or wife count on your word? How many promises have you broken already? For any marriage to be healthy and strong, the promises that the husband and wife have made to each other must be kept by both of them. On your wedding day you promise to be there for each other come rain, come shine and that no matter what happens you were never going to give up on each other. Andrew and Jackie like most couples thought marriage was just going to be a bed of rose, were you are in love forever without doing anything to sustain the relationship. Before they got married, they promised each other that nothing will ever separate them and that they will die for each other. Then they got married and could have enough of each other. Their promise to be there for one another seemed to be working, until Jackie got a promotion at work that required a substantial amount of travelling and in addition to travelling, she started bringing work home. The meant that most of the time even when she was at home, she was either on her laptop or checking her phone. Initially Andrew thought this was a temporal something, but it took a life of its own as time went on and Jackie became disengaged from the relationship and all she thought about was her work and the demands and the next promotion. No matter how much her husband tried to remind her of their promise to each other, Jackie did not care anymore. Let with nothing but broken promises Andrew is considering the unthinkable. Divorce!

Daily to do list

1) Read your why to each other.
2) Read the short daily devotional and meditate
3) Go out and exercise together
4) Focus on promises you made to each other and what that means to you and your relationship. Challenge each other during your exercise on ways to keep the promises you made to each other.
5) At the end of the day make a journal entry here on your observations and major takeaways.

_____

_____

_____

_____

_____

_____

_____

_____

_____

_____

_____

_____

Day 32

Thursday: Dependable

"Where would you be without friends? The people to pick you up when you need lifting? We come from homes far from perfect, so you end up almost parent and sibling to your friends – your own chosen family. There's nothing like a really loyal, dependable, good friend."
Nothing. Jennifer Aniston

The United States of America is the land of the brave free and the free. It is not uncommon to hear that you have to learn to pull yourself up by your bootstraps. There is a lot of talk about 'self-made" individuals who attribute their success to nobody but themselves. Most of the emphasis is on individual freedom and achievement. There is nothing wrong in being a strong individual and higher achiever. They can do it attitude is not evil in itself, but when you get married there is need for the two of you to learn how to work together. For the two of you to work together you have to create some dependability. There is nothing wrong in depending on each other and for you to be in need. We were created for relationship and part of the reason depression may be higher in affluent societies has to do with "the freedom" material things bring. People erroneously think that that material things will satisfy them, only to be disappointed because there is nothing that can replace a human touch.

Are you and you husband truly dependable on each other? Is there mutual give and take in your relationship, or each person is doing their own thing and on their own schedule? Both of you have to make it OK to depend on each other, for it takes two to tangle. This 90-day exercise challenge is a good opportunity for both of you to do just that. To become dependable is not something that just happens to you it is going to require intentionality on your part for this to become a reality. Your marriage needs both of you to be dependable if you want the marriage to be strong and for it to be divorce proof and meaningful at the same time.

Daily to do list

1) Read your why to each other.
2) Read the short daily devotional and meditate
3) Go out and exercise together
4) Focus on forgiveness and what that means to you and your relationship. Challenge each other during your exercise on ways to incorporate forgiveness in your marriage.
5) At the end of the day make a journal entry here on your observations and major takeaways.

_____

_____

_____

_____

_____

_____

_____

_____

_____

_____

_____

_____

_____

_____

Friday: Patience

*"Every great dream begins with a dreamer. Always remember,
you have within you the strength, the patience, and the passion
to reach for the stars to change the world."*
Harriet Tubman

When Luke and Rebeca were newly married, he dreaded the thought of both of them going out for any event. Luke was raised by a single dad and as far as he can remember, they always went to events on time and his father had instilled in him the importance of showing up on time. But he was not ready for what he was getting into. Because each time Luke and Rebeca are getting ready to go out for any event, Rebecca takes forever to get ready. Her not always getting ready on time has caused them to go late on many occasions and this does not sit well with Luke at all. Each time they are about to go out, Luke dreads the confrontation that will come up if he dares to suggest that time was running out and they were going to be late. You can see Luke pacing around the living room, agitated, and frustrated because Rebecca was trying on one blouse after the other and different shoes and handbags as well. It did not take long for Luke to realize that he was part of the problem because he was focusing only on the actions of Rebeca and not his impatience. He had thought about the fact that he was contributing to the misery that he was going through each time they planned to go out and has been trying to solve the problem wrongly. They have two children, that his wife has to get ready before they leave the house and it never occurred to him that he could help with the children, because Luke lacks the patience to get the children dressed.

Then one day it occurred to Luke that since his wife needs not less than an extra hour to get ready, it will be better to measure that extra hour is factored in the time he tells his wife they are going to leave the house. In addition to that he started helping with the children. Initially it was tough, but with time he got better and better at it.

Daily to do list

1) Read your why to each other.
2) Read the short daily devotional and meditate
3) Go out and exercise together
4) Focus on patience and what that means to you and your relationship. Challenge each other during your exercise on ways to incorporate patience in your marriage.
5) At the end of the day make a journal entry here on your observations and major takeaways.

_____

_____

_____

_____

_____

_____

_____

_____

_____

_____

_____

_____

_____

_____

Saturday: Longsuffering

"Our heavenly Father understands our disappointment, suffering, pain, fear, and doubt. He is always there to encourage our hearts and help us understand that He's sufficient for all of our needs. When I accepted this as an absolute truth in my life, I found that my worrying stopped."
Charles Stanley

Nobody wants to suffer or gets married to suffer. Why will anybody willingly subject themselves to suffering? Pam meet Jim during their freshman year in college and instantly feel in love with him. But they had a huge barrier, because Pam was from West Africa and Jim Caucasian. Back then it was a "taboo" for Caucasians to date people from African and there was no room for marriage. Pam and Jim were very aware of the challenge that was ahead of them and how difficult it was going to be for them if they continued hanging out and planning to get married. Jim's parents had sent him to college to get a business degree so that he will take over the family business after graduation. His mother could not stand the thought of having grandchildren that will not look "normal" and was adamantly opposed to the idea of Jim dating a girl from Africa. She expressed her displeasure by refusing to let Jim bring Pam home for Thanksgiving and vowed that Jim will not have access to the family business if he did not stop seeing Pam. Jim's father was on the same page with his wife and they cut all funds for Jim's schooling because he will not listen to them. This meant that Jim had to work and go to school. This is not something that he had been prepared for, because his parents were extremely wealthy and up to that point had taken care of all his needs. His friends could believe why he will let go of a comfortable life and guaranteed wealth for an African girl. Jim was determined to pay the price and suffer long for the love of his life. Instead of four years, it took him five to finish college and he had to go work for a different company with less pay and less benefits, because he had made a commitment to Pam. They eventually got married and after five years his parents came around.

Daily to do list

1) Read your why to each other.
2) Read the short daily devotional and meditate
3) Go out and exercise together
4) Focus on forgiveness and what that means to you and your relationship. Challenge each other during your exercise on ways to incorporate forgiveness in your marriage.
5) At the end of the day make a journal entry here on your observations and major takeaways.

_____

_____

_____

_____

_____

_____

_____

_____

_____

_____

_____

_____

_____

Day 35

Sunday: Tenacity

"Each season I find myself constantly inspired by 'The Biggest Loser' contestants. Their tenacity and willingness to learn new, healthy habits is tremendous and the results speak for themselves. I am honored to be part of such an inspiring program that helps inspire positive change in so many lives."
Curtis Stone

What keeps you going when everything else fails? You must have heard of marriages that have disintegrated and fallen apart because of irreconcilable differences. What that means is that the husband and wife are so set in their ways that there is no room for change and compromise. In other words, they hold to something that is more important than the marriage. One way to avoid falling into such a rot is to prioritize your marriage and place it above everything else. For this to happen you will need to be tenacious. There is a lot that is standing in the way of marriages today and it is going to take husbands and wives who have developed tenacity to stand up against all the distractions and opposition to marriage. Some of the opposition to marriage is subtle, for example people are working too hard and are so busy that there is little time left to nurture and take care of their marriages. Another issue is the fact that society has made divorce so easily available. The pursuit for material things is being celebrated at the expense of things that truly matter. Many say they are not pursuing material things, but their actions speak louder than their words. Show me where you spend your time and I will tell what is truly important to you. If your marriage is important you will put in the time, energy and effort that is necessary to keep it alive and vibrant. You neglect your marriage when you work too hard that there is nothing left to give when you come back home. You are so tired and easily irritated that it is becoming impossible to live under the same roof with you. Now is the time to push back against all the marriage destroyers and you will sure need to be tenacious to do that.

Daily to do list

1) Read your why to each other.
2) Read the short daily devotional and meditate
3) Take your weight and log it here: _____
4) Go out and exercise together
5) Focus on tenacity and what that means to you and your relationship. Challenge each other during your exercise on ways to incorporate tenacity in your marriage.
6) At the end of the day make a journal entry here on your observations and major takeaways.
7) Both of you have to compare notes, evaluate your progress, and make adjustments accordingly.

_____

_____

_____

_____

_____

_____

_____

_____

_____

_____

_____

Day 36

Monday: Sexual intercourse

*"We exist in this weirdly schizo culture, where sex is everywhere in the
media, and yet, at the same time, you don't sit down and have
a conversation about what you did in bed last night with your
friends. Despite the ubiquity of sex, it's still a taboo when
it comes to day-to-day conversation."*
Mary Roach

Can we talk about sec today? We are hoping that you are a legally
married couple with all the rights, responsibilities and privileges
that come with marriage. How is your sex life? What place does sex
occupy in your marriage? How often do you have good engaging
and fulfilling sex with one another? When was the last time you
introduced a new sex style in your relationship? I sex still exciting
and exhilarating as it was when you got married initially, or it is
something that you do these days out of necessity? Do you and
your partner talk freely, frankly, and sincerely about what your sex
needs are? Or you have some other means or person with whom you
meet your sextual needs? Sex is a gift from God for each married
couple to enjoy and there is nothing dirty or taboo about sex. In
fact, married couples should enjoy the best sex because they have the
right conditions for that to happen. Our hope is that during this 90-
day exercise challenge your sex life will be rekindled and the fire of
love will be lit and both of you will enjoy great sex again. There is a
direct connection between exercise and great sextual intercourse. We
discussed this in depth in our **book about the benefits** of couples
exercising together. If you have not read this book, we strongly
encourage you to get a couple and read it. Here is a summary of that

chapter on sex and exercise. When you exercise blood flows to your sex organs, you develop strong muscles, a stronger heart and release intimacy and feel good hormones. A combination of all these factors results in great sex. Do you want great sex in your marriage? You should exercise regular together with your husband or wife.

Daily to do list

1) Read your why to each other.
2) Read the short daily devotional and meditate
3) Go out and exercise together
4) Focus on sex and what that means to you and your relationship. Challenge each other during your exercise on ways to incorporate determination in your marriage.
5) At the end of the day make a journal entry here on your observations and major takeaways.

_____

_____

_____

_____

_____

_____

_____

_____

_____

_____

_____

_____

_____

_____

Tuesday: Thankfulness

*"A man who is eating or lying with his wife or preparing to go to sleep
in humility, thankfulness and temperance, is, by Christian standards,
in an infinitely higher state than one who is listening to Bach
or reading Plato in a state of pride."*
C. S. Lewis

A re you one of those couples who take each other for granted?
You seldomly say thank you, but is always quick to complain and
point out faults? Most relationships do not start like this, but time
has a way of making us to become complacent and unappreciative.
We tend to focus on what is not going right at the expense of all the
other good things that are going great in the marriage. This attitude
of ingratitude and taking each other for granted has the potential to
ruin any good marriage if allow to persist over time. Emily was so
excited with the surprise that she had put together for her husband
that she took the day off from work, just to make sure that everything
was right. She was trying to pull a big on him and was working so
hard to make sure that it remained a surprise. She had booked a
hotel room in another part of town for their one day get away. Her
husband saw the charge on their credit card and did not pay close
attention to what the charge was for, he concluded that Emily was
spending money unnecessarily and this made him mad. As he was
driving home from work that evening his mind was on the money
and how he was going to address his wife when he gets home. The
more he thought about it the angrier he got and by the time he drove
into the driveway he was boiling with anger and ready to explode.
Emily was excitedly waiting for the sound of his car to pull up in

the driveway to give him a big hug and kiss and was clueless about what was about to happen. Immediately her husband walked in she rushed towards him with wide opened arms, but her husband went into verbal assault immediately and ruined the whole evening.

Daily to do list

1) Read your why to each other.
2) Read the short daily devotional and meditate
3) Go out and exercise together
4) Focus on thankfulness and what that means to you and your relationship. Challenge each other during your exercise on ways to incorporate thankfulness in your marriage.
5) At the end of the day make a journal entry here on your observations and major takeaways.

_____

_____

_____

_____

_____

_____

_____

_____

_____

_____

_____

_____

_____

Wednesday: Fidelity

"When I talk about the importance of the institution of marriage, I think of the commitment and the significance of standing in front of those closest to you and promising fidelity to your partner 'til death do you part."
Mark Udall

Keeping your marriage vows is a cornerstone to the success of your marriage. There is no room for marital unfaithfulness. If you are cheating on your husband or wife now is the time to stop cheating and focus on building your marriage. Stolen water is sweet until it turns bitter in your stomach and you are focused to vomit. Unfortunately, modern technology has made it easier for husbands and wives to commit adultery. Some have decided to call it extra marital affairs, but that does not change the devastating consequences that are associated with adultery. In some cases, the husband or the wife may be committing emotional adultery, in that he or she has somebody that they are so emotionally connected that, each time they speak, they feel loved, accepted, and cherished. Because of the emotional high and satisfaction, the cheating partner gets from this "extra marital" association he or she is no longer connected to their married partner as they are supposed to. When they are on the phone or chatting with this particular person that they are now emotionally connected to them are nice, friendly, and put up their best face, but get angry, resentful, and feisty when talking with their husband or wife. They cheating partner is always extremely protective of their phone and does not allow anybody access to it. Does your husband or wife religiously protect their phone from you? Then there must be something going on that may eventually undermine your marriage. Most people do not start with the intention of committing emotional infidelity, but as time goes on, they just get deeper and deeper and in some cases it gets to the point where physical infidelity is committed. If you are caught up in such a trap now is the time to break free before it destroys your marriage.

Daily to do list

1) Read your why to each other.
2) Read the short daily devotional and meditate
3) Go out and exercise together
4) Focus on forgiveness and what that means to you and your relationship. Challenge each other during your exercise on ways to incorporate forgiveness in your marriage.
5) At the end of the day make a journal entry here on your observations and major takeaways.

_____

_____

_____

_____

_____

_____

_____

_____

_____

_____

_____

_____

Day 39

Thursday: Adultery

"The thing that alarms me is that there are so many clergymen who say that the so-called 'new morality' is all right. They say we're living in a new generation; let's be relevant, let's change God's law. Let's say that adultery is all right under certain circumstances; fornication's all right under certain circumstances. If it's 'meaningful.'"
Billy Graham

Adultery is a no no in any marriage and should be avoided at all cost. There is nothing more devastating for marriages than adultery. When a husband or wife chooses to commit adultery, they are willing breaking the foundation of their marriage and the consequences are devastating. Adultery is betrayal of the highest category and should not be treated lightly. The majority of married woman and men do like adultery for obvious reasons. Marriage is a covenant between two people and adultery breaks this convenient and the trust that is established between these two people. Adultery is so devastating that when asked to address the issue of divorce, Jesus had this to say; "But I tell you that anyone who divorces his wife, except for sexual immorality, makes her the victim of adultery, and anyone who marries a divorced woman commits adultery. The consequences of adultery are so dire that what God has put together adultery is the only thing that can put it asunder. That is why king Solomon who had 1000 wives gave the following warning concerning adultery;

But a man who commits adultery has no sense; whoever does so, destroys himself. Blows and disgrace are his lot, and his shame will never be wiped away. For jealousy arouses a husband's fury, and he will show no mercy when he takes revenge. He will not accept any compensation; he will refuse a bribe; however great it is. Proverbs 6:32-35

The long and the short of the matter is that stay away from adultery, because it will destroy you.

Daily to do list

1) Read your why to each other.
2) Read the short daily devotional and meditate
3) Go out and exercise together
4) Focus on adultery and what that means to you and your relationship. Challenge each other during your exercise on ways to prevent adultery in your marriage.
5) At the end of the day make a journal entry here on your observations and major takeaways.

_____

_____

_____

_____

_____

_____

_____

_____

_____

_____

_____

Day 40

Friday: Optimism

"The essence of optimism is that it takes no account of the present, but it is a source of inspiration, of vitality and hope where others have resigned; it enables a man to hold his head high, to claim the future for himself and not to abandon it to his enemy."
Dietrich Bonhoeffer

Kate and Jack got married immediately they graduated from high school and exactly one year after that their first son was born. After another year they had a second child this time a daughter. They had desired to have two children a boy and girl and their desire had been granted. Jack was having a good paying job and Kate was a stay at home mom. Everything was going well for them, then disaster stroked. Jack's company made a series of bad business decisions that impacted the profits of the company and they were forced to lay people off and Jack lost his job. When Jack got home that day, he got a phone call from his mother informing him that his father had been diagnosed with stage 4 cancer and the doctors had given him a few months to live. Jack was devasted because he was an only child and very close to his father. As they were still trying to figure out what to do, another phone call came from Kate's father, her mother was in a deadly motor accident and was on life support. A drunken driver had ramped in her car on the interstate highway and died on the spot. Kate and Jacob were devastated, and heart broken, it seemed the whole world was turning against them. Fortunately for them they were believers and people of faith and had to draw inspiration and strength from the following Bible verses;

And we know that God causes everything to work together for the good of those who love God and are called according to his purpose for them. Romans 8:28

"Do not be anxious about anything, but in every situation, by prayer and petition, with thanksgiving, present your requests to God. And the peace of God, which transcends all understanding, will guard your hearts and your minds in Christ Jesus."
Philippians 4:5-7

Daily to do list

1) Read your why to each other.
2) Read the short daily devotional and meditate
3) Go out and exercise together
4) Focus on optimism and what that means to you and your relationship. Challenge each other during your exercise on ways to incorporate optimism in your marriage.
5) At the end of the day make a journal entry here on your observations and major takeaways.

_____

_____

_____

_____

_____

_____

_____

_____

_____

_____

Day 41

Saturday: Unity

"Neither man nor woman is perfect or complete without the other.
Thus, no marriage or family, no ward or stake is likely to reach its full
potential until husbands and wives, mothers and fathers, men and
women work together in unity of purpose, respecting
and relying upon each other's strengths."
Sheri L. Dew

If you want to go far you will need to walk together and nothing
erodes unity in marriage more lack of trust. You have to work
together and walk together, and it will need unity for you to achieve
this. Unity is not something that just happens, it has to be developed
cultivated, nourished, and sustained over time. It will take hard
work, compromise and giving up of both of your "rights" to walk
in unity. The good news is that you are in a loving relationship and
have the capacity to achieve unity no matter what. The opposite
of unit is disunity and the consequences of are dire. Your marriage
will disintegrate and fall apart if there is no unity in your marriage.
You do not want what you have invested in for years to break and
fall apart, therefore it is in your best interest to ensure that there is
unity in your marriage. Listen to what Jesus Christ said about the
importance of unity and the danger of disunity;

"If a kingdom is divided against itself, it cannot stand.
If a house is divided against itself, it cannot stand."
Mark 3:25

There is a great need for unity in among husbands and wives if they want to stand up against the different forces that are acting against their marriage. You are never in a neutral state. Your marriage is either growing stronger or weaker, it is either improving or deteriorating. Therefore, presenting a united front as a husband and wife is your only hope of emerging victorious. One way to divorce proof your marriage is to walk and work in unity always.

Daily to do list

1) Read your why to each other.
2) Read the short daily devotional and meditate
3) Go out and exercise together
4) Focus on forgiveness and what that means to you and your relationship. Challenge each other during your exercise on ways to incorporate unity in your marriage.
5) At the end of the day make a journal entry here on your observations and major takeaways.

_____

_____

_____

_____

_____

_____

_____

_____

_____

_____

_____

_____

Day 42

Sunday: Harmony

"You are only afraid if you are not in harmony with yourself. People are afraid because they have never owned up to themselves."
Hermann Hesse

Do you know who you are? Do you know your strengths and weaknesses? There is none of us that can be extremely good at everything. That is why opposites attract so that they can complement each other. It is unfortunate that we spend a lot of time energy and money studying other subjects yet neglect the most important subject. You are the most important subject and it is crucial you study you if that has not already been done. When you understand who you are and accept your strengths and weaknesses, it will pave the way for you to achieve internal harmony. It is only after you have found harmony with yourself that you can have harmony with other people, especially your wife or husband.

The purpose of harmony is not sameness, it is to make the two of you walk together in synergy. When two people who are completely different from each other learn to accept their differences and complement each other something beautiful comes out of it. The interdependence that results from each one them completing each other is amazing. Take for example, in some marriages the husband may be scattered and disorganized, but his wife is organized and meticulous and is always trying to organize her husband. There is a tendency for this obvious difference between this husband and wife to be come a flash point. It should not be, because the goal of the wife in this case, should not be to "change" her husband to become organized and meticulous like her. It is tiring to keep organizing a disorganized room, but it is rewarding at the same time to be bringing something in the relationship that is highly need. In this the ability for the wife to be organized. If you carefully, the wife also has an area that she is struggling in and her husband maybe the one who is complementing her in that area.

Daily to do list

1) Read your why to each other.
2) Read the short daily devotional and meditate
3) Take your weight and log it here: _____
4) Go out and exercise together
5) Focus on determination and what that means to you and your relationship. Challenge each other during your exercise on ways to incorporate determination in your marriage.
6) At the end of the day make a journal entry here on your observations and major takeaways.
7) Both of you have to compare notes, evaluate your progress, and make adjustments accordingly.

_____

_____

_____

_____

_____

_____

_____

_____

_____

_____

Monday: Sincerity

"When you really need help, people will respond. Sincerity
means dropping the image facade and showing a willingness
to be vulnerable. Tell it the way it is, lumps and all. Don't worry
if your presentation isn't perfect; ask from your heart. Keep
it simple, and people will open up to you."
Jack Canfield

Political correctness is evil and will destroy the foundation of any marriage. It is sad that many people in the name of love do not do what is right for their loved ones. The reason is that they love their comfort and acceptance more than the person the supposedly say they love. How can you let your loved one continue driving on a road you know is taking them down a cliff that will cause their death? Let us put it this way, there is a road that suddenly ends at the top of a cliff and your love one tells you they want to get on that road for a night drive. You will firmly tell them not to and if they insist you are going to do all within your power to ensure that they do not get on that road. You may escalate your intervention if they continue to insist that they do not believe you and will get on that road. Nobody is going to fault you to doing all within your power to prevent your loved one from certain death. When you succeed in dissuading them from this death path, everybody will hail you as a hero. But why is it that we shy behind and hide under the disguise of, "I don't want to judge anybody" when our loved ones are engaged in destructive behaviors? We do not like the confrontation and possible rejection that may result when we try to intervene. Therefore, we sooth our consciences by becoming politically correct. We stop being sincere and tell them white lies. Telling people what they want to and like to hear when you know that it will not help them in the long run is wickedness. Of what use is information that will not help your loved one's situation to change or improve? It is imperative for any husband and wife to be sincere, honest, and truthful to each other.

Daily to do list

1) Read your why to each other.
2) Read the short daily devotional and meditate
3) Go out and exercise together
4) Focus on sincerity and what that means to you and your relationship. Challenge each other during your exercise on ways to incorporate sincerity in your marriage.
5) At the end of the day make a journal entry here on your observations and major takeaways.

_____

_____

_____

_____

_____

_____

_____

_____

_____

_____

_____

_____

_____

_____

Day 44

Tuesday: Inspiration

*"Nature is my manifestation of God. I go to
nature every day for inspiration in the day's
work. I follow in building the principles which
nature has used in its domain."*
Frank Lloyd Wright

Inspiration means different things to different people, but in the context of marriage it has to do with innovation, creativity, and vitality. What is it that makes you come to life? In other words what makes your marriage come to life? Inspiration is very necessary because without it you will die. Marriages also need inspiration because they marriage will become stagnant and eventually a die if there is no inspiration. You have to keep the inspiration alive. What is that thing that brought you together? What did you see in each other when you met for the first time and what prompted you to get married to each other? Once more king Solomon has some powerful words here for each husband and wife to consider;

*"Drink water from your own cistern, running water from your own
well. Should your springs overflow in the streets, your streams of water
in the public squares. Let them be yours alone, never to be shared with
strangers. May your fountain be blessed, and may you rejoice in the wife
of your youth. A loving doe, a graceful deer—may her breasts satisfy
you always, may you ever be intoxicated with her love. Why, my son, be
intoxicated with another man's wife? Why embrace
the bosom of a wayward woman?"*
Proverbs 5: 15-20

Daily to do list

1) Read your why to each other.
2) Read the short daily devotional and meditate
3) Go out and exercise together
4) Focus on inspiration and what that means to you and your relationship. Challenge each other during your exercise on ways to incorporate inspiration in your marriage.
5) At the end of the day make a journal entry here on your observations and major takeaways.

_____

_____

_____

_____

_____

_____

_____

_____

_____

_____

_____

_____

_____

_____

_____

_____

_____

Wednesday: Transparency

"I think the currency of leadership is transparency. You've got to be truthful. I don't think you should be vulnerable every day, but there are moments where you've got to share your soul and conscience with people and show them who you are, and not be afraid of it."
Howard Schultz

It is recorded in Genesis chapter one that Adam and Eve were naked, but not ashamed. Transparency has to do with being "naked" and not ashamed. How naked are you? Are you hiding things from each other? Do you cover up your weaknesses and put up false persona? Are who you say you are, or you live a double life? It takes more energy to live an opaque life than being transparent and an open. One of the foundational stones of a strong and lasting marriage is transparency. You have to say what you are thinking and mean what you are saying. It is unacceptable to have a secondary life that is hidden from your husband or wife. How can you in good faith be carrying out capital intensive projects and investments without the knowledge of your wife or husband? The killers of transparency are fear and ignorance. Most fear is rooted in ignorance. That is why you need to deal with the fear in the right way in most cases getting the right information will drive fear away. Now is the time to remove all the barriers that making it difficult for you to truly connect with your husband or wife. There is some amount of venerability that is associated with transparency and many people do not like to be venerable. The result is that they sacrifice transparency on the altar of fear. Intimacy is enhanced by being transparent and open. This is an imperative in any marriage that has prospects of lasting long. As you and your husband and wife will spend some time exercising together you will have enough time to talk and open up to each other in ways that you might have up till now. DO not allow fear to hold you back for truly engaging each other and being transparent in the process.

Daily to do list

1) Read your WHY to each other.
2) Read the short daily devotional and meditate
3) Go out and exercise together
4) Focus on transparency and what that means to you and your relationship. Challenge each other during your exercise on ways to incorporate transparency into your marriage.
5) At the end of the day make a journal entry here on your observations and major takeaways.

_____

_____

_____

_____

_____

_____

_____

_____

_____

_____

_____

_____

_____

Thursday: Honesty

"My parents taught me honesty, truth, compassion, kindness and how to care for people. Also, they encouraged me to take risks, to boldly go. They taught me that the greatest danger in life is not taking the adventure."
Brian Blessed

Let us be honest, nobody wants to hang around dishonest people no matter what. We know the devastating consequences of dishonesty. Zack was the ideal husband because he was from a good home, had a good college degree and an excellent paying job. When you talk with him you leave with the impression that he will be an excellent person to spend the rest of your wife with. No wonder Emily fell for his charm and charisma when she met him at a country club event. Soon after that they got married before long were expecting their first child. During their courtship Emily had not suspected anything unusual about Zack, but a few months to the birth of their first child, she started noticing some unusual behaviors. For example, Zack started coming home late after work. In the beginning he will coming an hour late, then it became two hours and eventually Emily will go to bed without him coming back and only wake up in the morning and see lying by her side. When she tried to ask him what was going on, initially blamed an important project that had been placed in charge and the deadline was fast approaching. This had made sense initially and the prospect of a promotion at the end of the year calmed Emily a little. She reasoned that they were expecting a baby and she was going to stop working and an increase in her husband's salary was going to be God sent. But when Zack started coming home after midnight

Emily became suspicious that something was wrong, and Zack was not telling her the truth. He fears where confirmed when he came him one night and his breath was smelling with alcohol and unknown to Zack there was lipstick on the collar of his shirt. Zack was having an affair with one of his colleagues at work and had been hiding it from his wife. Each day after work they will go out for happy hour and pass through her house before Zack drove home.

Daily to do list

1) Read your WHY to each other.
2) Read the short daily devotional and meditate
3) Go out and exercise together
4) Focus on honesty and what that means to you and your relationship. Challenge each other during your exercise on ways to honesty forgiveness into your marriage.
5) At the end of the day make a journal entry here on your observations and major takeaways.

_____

_____

_____

_____

_____

_____

_____

_____

_____

_____

Friday: Charity

"Men lose all the material things they leave behind them in this world, but they carry with them the reward of their charity and the alms they give. For these, they will receive from the Lord the reward and recompense they deserve."
Francis of Assisi

When the word charity is mentioned many people think about starving and malnourished children in some third world country. For some people the word charity evokes felling of despair and haplessness. Take the case of Dacka, who was born and raised in a refugee camp in east Africa and was eventually brought to the United States of America by a refugee resettlement agency. The conditions in the camp where Dacka was born were so bad that, even after he arrived the United States of America it took him months to knock of the stench that was hanging over the camp from his subconscious mind. They were 100 percent dependent on foreign aid, and the rations were usually not enough for everyone, especially when your parents are sick and lack the stamina to stand in the long lines on the days the food is distributed. It was truly the survival of the fittest in the camp and many did not survive. Even now Dacka wonders how he survived.

Your marriage is not about to collapse nor are you starving. If you are reading this the probability that you are doing well is high. That said, we want you to take a different look at charity and how it can improve your marriage. Many people give to strangers, help outsiders, and show kindness and tolerance to other people, but become vicious and unbearing when it concerns their loved ones. You must have heard that "charity begins at home." If you have not now is the time for both of you to practice some charity in your marriage and be a source of healing, encouragement and blessing to each other. Volunteer to be good to another.

Daily to do list

1) Read your why to each other.
2) Read the short daily devotional and meditate
3) Go out and exercise together
4) Focus on charity and what that means to you and your relationship. Challenge each other during your exercise on ways to incorporate charity in your marriage.
5) At the end of the day make a journal entry here on your observations and major takeaways.

_____

_____

_____

_____

_____

_____

_____

_____

_____

_____

_____

_____

_____

Day 48

Saturday: Discernment

"As soldiers need not only courage but tactics also, so does
a philosopher need not only courage and philosophy
but discernment also, to tell what his right time of
dying is – so that he neither seek it nor flee it."
Apollonius of Tyana

Reading in-between the lines requires more than head knowledge and it can make the difference between a good marriage and a great marriage. The ability to be discerning will set your marriage apart, by moving it from the natural to the supernatural. It will ensure that you are always a step ahead of whatever is happening. It is always tempting to settle for the normal, the usual and the predictable. The ability to differentiate between what is heard, seen and what truly is will make huge difference in your marriage. Take for example you may come back from work and your wife greets you with less enthusiasm. In you are discerning you will look for an appropriate amount to dig deeper and figure out what is going on with her. Unfortunately, many undiscerning husbands will go into the attack mode and escalate the situation out of proportion. One thing will to lead to another and a few minutes into the argument the breaks out both of you will be on each other's throats. This is a situation that could have been avoided if both of you were discerning enough.

Most of the arguments, fights and quarrels in marriages will be avoided if discernment is utilized by both husbands and wives. The good news is that everybody can learn to be discerning. It will not just happen, but you will have to put in some hard work and let go of your own biases, stereotypes, past hurts, resentment, and preconceived notions. It is going to take discipline on your part to read between the lines and arrive the right conclusions.

Daily to do list

1) Read your why to each other.
2) Read the short daily devotional and meditate
3) Go out and exercise together
4) Focus on discernment and what that means to you and your relationship. Challenge each other during your exercise on ways to incorporate discernment in your marriage.
5) At the end of the day make a journal entry here on your observations and major takeaways.

_____

_____

_____

_____

_____

_____

_____

_____

_____

_____

_____

_____

_____

Day 49

Sunday: Wisdom

"Knowledge comes, but wisdom lingers. It may not be difficult to store up in the mind a vast quantity of facts within a comparatively short time, but the ability to form judgments requires the severe discipline of hard work and the tempering heat of experience and maturity."
Calvin Coolidge

The fear of the Lord is the begging of wisdom. To fear God is to hate evil. We know evil when we see it and when we experience it as well. You are going to need a lot of wisdom to navigate the complexities that are associated with marriage. Many people take if for granted that they are married and just assume that it is going to work out because they are living together. Some reason that because they have "fallen in love" all is going to be well. But wake up one day and all the love is gone and all they think about is separating and going in two different directions. Others who do not separate stay in the same house but are not together, because each person is doing their own thing. We are living in a generation that is saturated with a lot of information, but wisdom is scare. There are some many excellent marriage seminars, teachings, books, tapes etc., but the divorce rate has been growing steadily. The simple reason is that head knowledge is not good enough. You may claim how much you know and can even talk about it passionately and with conviction, but if you do not act on what you say you know, nothing will change. Wisdom is knowing that it is not enough to read a book, listen to a good message, you have to apply the information that you have gathered. If you are wise you will do what you know you are supposed to be doing.

Daily to do list

1) Read your why to each other.
2) Read the short daily devotional and meditate
3) Take your weight and log it here_____
4) Go out and exercise together
5) Focus on wisdom and what that means to you and your relationship. Challenge each other during your exercise on ways to wisdom determination in your marriage.
6) At the end of the day make a journal entry here on your observations and major takeaways.
7) Both of you have to compare notes, evaluate your progress and make adjustments accordingly.

_____
_____
_____
_____
_____
_____
_____
_____
_____
_____
_____
_____
_____
_____
_____

Monday: Character

"Character cannot be developed in ease and quiet. Only through experience of trial and suffering can the soul be strengthened, ambition inspired, and success achieved."
Helen Keller

Are you a person of character? What distinguishes you from others? Are you somebody who stands out in a crowd or you go along with the flow? There are too few people of character, no wonder our marriages are disintegrating at an alarming rate. Talk is cheap, but it takes time hard work, sweat and toil to become a person of character. Unfortunately, in this feel good generation many are on the road of list resistance and are not developing the mental toughness and grit that is needed for strong character development. Your marriage is the most important thing you will ever do and you should defend it, fight for it and stand up against and opposition. There is no short cut to character development, you will have to roll up your sleeves get into the trenches of life and dig hard. Many of the current inconveniences and discomforts that you are experiencing because you are married are supposed to be helping get you into shape. Marriage does two things for you and both things occur concurrently. These two things are character development and pleasure, with the former being more important than the later. But the more you develop your character the more pleasure you will get out of your marriage. Therefore, focus on developing your character and all the pleasure you desire will eventually follow. It takes character to be patient, kind, loving, and persevere. Many people give up to soon because they lack what it takes to wait. They have not developed the tenacity and mental fortitude that is necessary for them to endure to the end. You case is going to be different because you have made a commitment to finish this 90-day challenge after 50 days you are still in.

Daily to do list

1) Read your why to each other.
2) Read the short daily devotional and meditate
3) Go out and exercise together
4) Focus on character and what that means to you and your relationship. Challenge each other during your exercise on ways to incorporate character development in your marriage.
5) At the end of the day make a journal entry here on your observations and major takeaways.

_____

_____

_____

_____

_____

_____

_____

_____

_____

_____

_____

_____

_____

Tuesday: Attitude

*"Develop an attitude of gratitude, and give thanks for everything
that happens to you, knowing that every step forward is a step toward
achieving something bigger and better than your current situation."*
Brian Tracy

Attitude is everything! There is no place where attitude is more important than in marriage. The quality of your marriage is directly proportional to your attitude. Some have said, "your attitude will determine your altitude." In other words, how far and how high you fly is based on your attitude. We are going to add here that how much your marriage will flourish is dependent on your attitude. Nothing spoils a marriage and kills romance and intimacy like a bad attitude. If there is anything that all married husbands and wives have to avoid, a bad attitude is number one on the list. For one of the most disheartening and uncomfortable things to do is living under the same roof with somebody with a bad attitude. If you have a nagging, complaining and negative attitude, you are going to make those around you miserable, especially you husband or wife. This issue of having a bad attitude is not new, a few thousand years ago King Solomon wrote the following,

*"It's better to stay outside on the roof of your
house than to live inside with a nagging wife."*
Proverbs, 21:9 (Contemporary English Version)

A bad attitude will drive your partner way and force them to make some drastic decisions. This unfortunate situation can be avoided if both husband and wife develop an attitude of gratitude. You should never take each other for granted and make it a daily habit to count your blessings and name them one by one. You will be amazed by how much blessed you are.

Daily to do list

1) Read your why to each other.
2) Read the short daily devotional and meditate
3) Go out and exercise together
4) Focus on forgiveness and what that means to you and your relationship. Challenge each other during your exercise on ways to incorporate forgiveness in your marriage.
5) At the end of the day make a journal entry here on your observations and major takeaways.

_____

_____

_____

_____

_____

_____

_____

_____

_____

_____

_____

_____

_____

Day 52

Wednesday: Affection

"So many of us have loved ones and people we really care about, and the only time we show affection is when they are gone. I have preached at funerals, and you see loved ones who didn't even say hello to dear ones when they were alive. Give them hugs, kisses while they are alive and need it."
George Foreman

We have talked about taking each other granted already and will mention that again because it is extremely important. Any health marriage that will last long must incorporate affection in it. To be affectionate is going to take some intentionality and hard work. Yes, hard work! Many marriages are on the brink of collapse because the husband and wife have been waiting for something good to happen to them. The reality is that nothing good will happen, if they do not do anything. Instead their marriage will deteriorate. This myth of "falling in love" has ruined many lives, because many people allow their feelings to lead them. No wonder a couple that professed they were so much in love will suddenly be at odds with each other to the extent that divorcing is the only option and the one of the common reasons is irreconcilable differences. What happened to love? Does love not to cover a multitude of sins? Love is supposed to believe all, bear all, and suffer long. It seems many people have different definitions of what love is.

It is the responsibility of both husband and wife to ensure that there is affection in their marriage. Learning your husband or wife's love language and speaking it is an important component of showing affection. Never assume anything, it is in the best interest of the welfare of your marriage to ensure that you know what the other person needs. Bringing in the flowers, giving hugs, saying I love you and being gentle the way you talk to each other is good. Do not wait for your husband or wife to die before you tell them how much they meant to you. Let them hear while they are alive.

Daily to do list

1) Read your why to each other.
2) Read the short daily devotional and meditate
3) Go out and exercise together
4) Focus on affection and what that means to you and your relationship. Challenge each other during your exercise on ways to incorporate affection in your marriage.
5) At the end of the day make a journal entry here on your observations and major takeaways.

_____

_____

_____

_____

_____

_____

_____

_____

_____

_____

_____

Thursday: Competition

"Your competition is not other people but the time you kill, the ill will you create, the knowledge you neglect to learn, the connections you fail to build, the health you sacrifice along the path, your inability to generate ideas, the people around you who don't support and love your efforts, and whatever god you curse for your bad luck."
James Altucher

You did not get married to compete with each other or with other married couples. The focus should never be on trying to become like the Joneses down the street. You should focus on being all you were created to be. When both the husband and wife becoming students of personal growth and development their marriage will automatically grow because they will get better and better with each passing day. The better you will make a better mate. It is imperative that you remain a student and keep learning. There are too many good resources that will help you grow, spiritually, physically, financially, emotionally etc. It is not enough to earn a degree; you have to continue learning after you graduate. Unfortunately, many people do not read at all. The few that read, do not apply the knowledge that is acquired. No wonder we are saturated with information, yet most of our marriage are ending up in divorce and the obesity rate is on the rise globally. The prison population is on the rise as well. There is no point acquiring knowledge and not using it. Therefore, the true competition that you are up against is what you do with your time and not where other people are or what they are doing. It is a waste of time energy and resources to focus on what other people are doing and neglect what is within your own power to do and improve your marriage and circumstances. For example, make it a habit to can read a book together.

Daily to do list

1) Read your why to each other.
2) Read the short daily devotional and meditate
3) Go out and exercise together
4) Focus on competition and what that means to you and your relationship. Challenge each other during your exercise on ways to incorporate competition in your marriage.
5) At the end of the day make a journal entry here on your observations and major takeaways.

_____

_____

_____

_____

_____

_____

_____

_____

_____

_____

_____

_____

_____

_____

_____

_____

Day 54

Friday: Compliments

"I really think that you have to find a partner that compliments you and is somebody that pushes you and is better at some things than you are, so they can push you to improve yourself as a person."
Ashton Kutcher

Anyi had been married to Ekong for over 20 years and they have eaten out for 19 of those years. Right now, they are in some financial difficulties because of some unfortunate financial decisions that they have made. They decided to see a financial advisor on the way forward and she told them to draw a budget and figure out ways to cut back on their expenses. One of the areas to cut back that could save them a lot of money was eating out. They were having two children and have been spending close to a third of their income on eating out. When the idea of cutting back on eating out was suggested, Anyi fought back vigorously and rightfully so. When they had just gotten married, she was so excited to fix meals for her young husband. Unfortunately, each time he came home he will complain about the food, from there is no salt to too much salt, no oil too much oil etc. Each time he will end up ordering something else to eat and at times will go out to to eat. Ekong reasoned that he could afford to eat whatever he wanted and will not be "punished" by his wife's poor cooking. He never complimented Anyi for almost a year despite the fact that she did all she could do accommodate his demands and complains. At the end of a year of eating her cooking by herself, Anyi got tired and joined her us to eat out and other meals. They started having children and it became a convenient thing to do, then the financial disaster hit and now they are having a hard time digging their way out of the mess.

It is a must for husbands and wives to complement each other and to do that regularly and consistently. Why do you compliment the chefs in the restaurants that you eat, but never compliment your wife or husband when they prepare a meal for the family?

Daily to do list

1) Read your why to each other.
2) Read the short daily devotional and meditate
3) Go out and exercise together
4) Focus on forgiveness and what that means to you and your relationship. Challenge each other during your exercise on ways to incorporate forgiveness in your marriage.
5) At the end of the day make a journal entry here on your observations and major takeaways.

_____

_____

_____

_____

_____

_____

_____

_____

_____

_____

_____

_____

Saturday: Praise

"Employees who report receiving recognition and praise within the last seven days show increased productivity, get higher scores from customers, and have better safety records. They're just more engaged at work."
Tom Rath

Stop taking each other for granted. How often do you say thank you after you have sex with your husband or wife? Do you just think it is supposed to happen and has happen and everything is cool? When was the last time you thank you husband for taking out the trash? How often do you thank your wife for fixing the dinner or packing your lunch? What about taking care of the children, running errands, and ensuring that all the bills are paid on time? We all crave for recognition, reward and praise at work, but when we come home, we expect to work hard but not get reward, praised and promoted? The reason is that we take each other for granted and this is wrong. You did not get married to a house maid, nor did you get married for a handyman. Both of you got married to complement each other and help each other become all you were created to be. Therefore, it is not proper to take for granted what you do for one another on a daily basis. It is important to say thank daily, frequently, and unfailingly. Try it and see how much it will improve your marriage. You may be wondering if saying thank you will not appear to mean that you are not being sincere. You can never go wrong with saying thank you from the depth of your heart. Make it a point of duty to say thank you to your husband or wife when you get up each morning. Praise them for sharing their life with you and for going through the thick and thin with you. Praise your wife for putting their live on the line for all the children you have been blessed with. Do not say that you have said it once and that is enough. Just like taking a bath and brushing your teeth daily, it is crucial for you to apply a daily dose of praise on each other.

Daily to do list

1) Read your why to each other.
2) Read the short daily devotional and meditate
3) Go out and exercise together
4) Focus on forgiveness and what that means to you and your relationship. Challenge each other during your exercise on ways to incorporate forgiveness in your marriage.
5) At the end of the day make a journal entry here on your observations and major takeaways.

_____

_____

_____

_____

_____

_____

_____

_____

_____

_____

_____

_____

_____

_____

Sunday: Rest

*"Sleeping is like meditation: it's good to rest the body
but also to shut the mind down for a bit."*
Anthony Joshua

We are too busy and do not take enough time to rest and recover from the stress if modern living. Taking time off to rest is not a luxury, it is extremely essential and any couple that wants their marriage to be strong and for it to last long MUST take rest seriously. There is no substitute to resting. Unfortunately, most husbands and wives are on the move all the time and sleep deprivation is one of the calamities of our time. Without proper sleep and the quality of life is negatively impacted. It is not uncommon to become easy irritated and agitated with the least provocation because you lack rest. There is another dimension of rest that is even more crucial, that is internal rest of the spirit. If you have not found rest for your soul and spirit, external rest alone will not suffice. Jesus Christ of Nazareth said,

"Come to me, all you who are weary and burdened, and I will give you rest. Take my yoke upon you and learn from me, for I am gentle and humble in heart, and you will find rest for your souls. For my yoke is easy and my burden is light." Matthew 11:28-30 New International Version (NIV)

What are some of the burdens that you are carrying? What load is making you afraid of the future and regretful of the past? If you turn over the burden to Jesus Christ, He will give you rest.

Daily to do list

1) Read your why to each other.
2) Read the short daily devotional and meditate
3) Take your weight and log it here_____
4) Go out and exercise together
5) Focus on determination and what that means to you and your relationship. Challenge each other during your exercise on ways to incorporate determination in your marriage.
6) At the end of the day make a journal entry here on your observations and major takeaways.
7) Both of you have to compare notes, evaluate your progress, and make adjustments accordingly.

_____

_____

_____

_____

_____

_____

_____

_____

_____

_____

_____

_____

_____

_____

_____

Day 57

Monday: Assurance

"In my experience, all Americans - Republicans, Democrats, and
everyone in between - want roughly the same thing: an assurance that
if they work hard, they can create a better life for themselves and their
families. They want to feel safe in their communities and
secure in their future."
Todd Young

Can you husband count on you? How about your wife, can she depend on you? If you want to depend your marriage, there must be some assurances. Now you go about it will depend on who you are. It is important that you be a person of your word. When you say something, you must follow through with it. Nobody gets married to be abandoned on the way. Everybody gets married hoping that the marriage will last till death parts them. Can each of you assure each other of this? This is going to take both of you working together and prioritizing your marriage. You cannot afford not to create an environment that is permeated with assurance that you are going to be there for each other. It is going to take more than signing the marriage certificate and taking marriage vows. You will have to follow through on the promises that you made to each other in the beginning. Creating an environment of assurance in your marriage can be done by you reminding each other of your commitment to be there for each other come rain come shine. Make it a daily habit to get your husband or wife into your arms look them straight in their eyes and tell that that you will always be there for them and that you will never leave them no matter what. You can also add that you will take care of them and share whatever blessings that come your way with them. Marriages are not only destroyed by hard times; success can also torpedo a marriage if the husband and wife does not know how to handle success. What you say often is eventually going to influence your believe system and your actions. What you act upon is going to determine the outcome that you get. Assure each other to be there for one another.

Daily to do list

1) Read your why to each other.
2) Read the short daily devotional and meditate
3) Go out and exercise together
4) Focus on forgiveness and what that means to you and your relationship. Challenge each other during your exercise on ways to incorporate forgiveness in your marriage.
5) At the end of the day make a journal entry here on your observations and major takeaways.

_____

_____

_____

_____

_____

_____

_____

_____

_____

_____

_____

_____

Tuesday: Resentment

"Resentment is like drinking poison and waiting
for the other person to die."
Saint Augustine

In every marriage there it is not uncommon for the husband and wife to hurt each other. If this is not happening, then these two people are not humans. The challenge is how to mitigate these hurts and what to do when they hurt each other. There are two responses, forgiveness and unforgiveness. To forgive is the higher ground and those who walk on that road are strong, wise and have understood that letting go brings more in return. It may not make sense in the immediate but in the long run the reward is huge. Unfortunately, many refuses to walk on the high road, but choose the low road of unforgiveness. They justify this by holding to their pain and hurt. They like to show people how badly they have been bruised and how painful they feel. Most of the time those listening to them give them a sympathetic ear and make them feel good and justified for holding to the pain, hurt and anger. There is no other benefit to holding onto the pain and hurt. The smartest and wisest thing to do is to forgive and let go of the pain and hurt. If you fail to forgive, you are going to develop resentment. The danger with resentment is that it is a ticking time bomb, that will torpedo your marriage when you least expect. Nobody wants to step on a landmine. When you harbor resentment in your marriage you are planting landmines that will blow your husband or wife into pieces when they step on them. Your will reach out of proposition to the least trigger because the pain and hurt have been adequately dealt with.

As Saint Augustine eloquently put it, "Resentment is like drinking poison and waiting for the other person to die." Get rid of the root of bitterness and let go of resentment, for it will poison you and not your partner. But you say be thinking that you will lose something for letting go of your pain and hurt, well you will gain, peace, joy, hope, happiness, and better health above a great marriage. So, get rid of any resentment in your heart now.

Daily to do list

1) Read your why to each other.
2) Read the short daily devotional and meditate
3) Go out and exercise together
4) Focus on forgiveness and what that means to you and your relationship. Challenge each other during your exercise on ways to incorporate forgiveness in your marriage.
5) At the end of the day make a journal entry here on your observations and major takeaways.

_____

_____

_____

_____

_____

_____

_____

_____

_____

_____

_____

_____

Day 59

Wednesday: Support

"I want someone who is my partner in life. Who supports me, and I support her. I can share all my experiences in life with her, and she can share hers back with me. Not only do we love each other, but we accept, embrace, nurture, and care for each other."
Tucker Max

Are you supportive? Can you husband or wife rely on you? There is a great need for every husband and wife to be a source of support for each other. You need to be strong enough for your husband or wife to lean on you, because if you are not strong enough you will not be able to support them when they need your help. Sooner or later you are going to hit a hard patch and there is nothing more comforting than somebody who loves and supports you. There will be a big need for a shoulder for you to lean on a n cry and your husband and wife should offer that shoulder when the time comes. Support is not only needed when the going gets tough, it is needed when new ideas come up. Many husband or wives are the first people to kill any new ideas that come up. They do not allow enough time to process the information before ruling it out and shooting the idea. Nothing is more discouraging than discouragement from your husband or wife. That is why it is crucial for each husband and wife to learn how to be supportive when the need arises. This can be done through your words and actions that you take or do not take. It is tempting to allow past experiences to cloud your judgment, all must be done by you to resist this and ensure that you use discernment to offer the right advice. If in doubt do not say anything than say something that will destroy instead of build. At times all you need to be supportive is just to listen and say nothing. Make sure that you are approachable, and your husband or wife can come to you anytime they need support. Who else do you think is equipped to carry out this crucial function in your marriage? If you do not offer the support that your husband or wife needs, who will?

Daily to do list

1) Read your why to each other.
2) Read the short daily devotional and meditate
3) Go out and exercise together
4) Focus on forgiveness and what that means to you and your relationship. Challenge each other during your exercise on ways to incorporate forgiveness in your marriage.
5) At the end of the day make a journal entry here on your observations and major takeaways.

_____

_____

_____

_____

_____

_____

_____

_____

_____

_____

_____

_____

_____

Thursday: Words

"Good words cool more than cold water."
John Ray

You must have heard that that "words do not kill," This is partly true, bad words are deadly and no marriage no matter how strong it is can withstand a barrage of bad and negative words. Have you ever said something and wish you had not? When words come out, they cannot be taken back. Therefore, we must guard our mouths and ensure that we think before we speak. King Solomon of old made the following statement about the power of the tongue, "The power of life and death lies in the tongue." Each time you open your mouth to speak, you are either speaking life or death, encouragement or discouragement, peace, or terror You get the point! Words become even more deadly among husbands and wives because they are living in close proximity with each other and the words spoken are not easily forgotten. Therefore, the husband and wife have to be aware of this and chose their words carefully. There is no place for demeaning, insulting and degrading words in a marriage. Instead of being mean with your words, chose words of encouragement, hope, peace, and joy. It is easier to be negative than positive, but it is more profitable to be positive and to use positive words more often.

How you talk to each other speaks volumes of the health of your relationship. Unhealthy and abusive marriages are characterized by negative words that keep pushing the marriage on a downward spiral of hopelessness, despair, and eventually destruction. Do not use words lightly when talking to each other. You must resist the temptation of using words to batter, belittle and put down each other. Avoid using your words to hurt, instead let your words, build, heal, restore comfort, and bring hope. Both of you will have to learn how to consistently use the right words when you speak to each other. At times it is better to not say anything, than speak hurt.

Daily to do list

1) Read your why to each other.
2) Read the short daily devotional and meditate
3) Go out and exercise together
4) Focus on words and what that means to you and your relationship. Challenge each other during your exercise on ways to incorporate the right words in your marriage.
5) At the end of the day make a journal entry here on your observations and major takeaways.

_____

_____

_____

_____

_____

_____

_____

_____

_____

_____

_____

_____

_____

Friday: Listen

"When a woman is talking to you, listen to
what she says with her eyes."
Victor Hugo

It is more difficult to listen than to speak. This is not an understatement and every couple that loves their marriage and want to keep it growing healthier and strong must take this seriously. They must understand the importance of listening and the role it plays in fostering robust marriages. Have you ever heard your wife or husband asking you if you are listening to them in the middle of a conversation? The obvious answer is always "yes I am listening". But the truth is that you were sitting there, but not listening. It takes more than being there to listen. There is something called active listening and it is imperative that all husbands and wives learn how to be active listeners. Many good books have been written on this subject and if you want to explore it more, you just need to search active listening on amazon or check with your local library. That said, it is important to remember that one way to actively listen is to avoid thinking about what to say while the other person is speaking. You should be focusing on hearing what they are saying instead working on the response in your mind. It is imperative that you just listen and soak in what the other person is saying. You goal is connecting with them and hearing not only what their mouth is saying, but what their eyes, heart, body, and soul is saying. It is going to take some degree of intentionality, focus and self-discipline on your part for this to happen. The tendency for the majority of us is to turn a deaf ear and draw conclusions and determine what we have to say before the other person finish speaking. 90% of all the communication problems in marriages will go away if the husband and wife learn how to be active listeners. Nothing will bring you closer more than knowing that your husband or wife truly hears you when you talk to them. Most of the time the wife or husband is not looking for a solution, but somebody to listen to them and share whatever they are going through. Start listening actively today if you are already doing so.

Daily to do list

1) Read your why to each other.
2) Read the short daily devotional and meditate
3) Go out and exercise together
4) Focus on listening and what that means to you and your relationship. Challenge each other during your exercise on ways to incorporate active listening in your marriage.
5) At the end of the day make a journal entry here on your observations and major takeaways.

_____

_____

_____

_____

_____

_____

_____

_____

_____

_____

_____

Saturday: Silence

"It is better wither to be silent, or to say things of more value than silence. Sooner throw a pearl at hazard than an idle or useless word; and do not say a little in many words, but a great deal in a few."
Pythagoras

You must have heard that "silence is golden." This is not the same has "giving the silent treatment" when one partner decides to use silence to punish the other. This type of silence has no place in a healthy marriage and should be avoided as the plague, for it is extremely destructive and hampers intimacy and good communication. But there is a place for silence in a marriage. Because at times it is better not to say anything than speak words that are destructive and hurtful. Job is one of the people that many of us know about his troubles. He lost all his children and investments on a single day and in addition to that was stricken by a dreadful disease and left to die. As the account goes, his three close friends showed up to comfort him. When they arrived Job's, situation was so pathetic that for a week they just sat in silence for lack of words to comfort their beloved friend. After waiting for seven days, his friend broke their silence and all they did from that pint onward was to blame Job for being the cause of his problems. According to two of these friends Job must have sinned and done something bad for him to be punished in this manner. Only one of the friends had a different take. How I wish Job's friends just remined silent, they would have avoided bring the wrath of God on them as they did, because their words were out of the will of God. There are times in your marriage that you MUST not speak, no matter how urgent the urge to speak may be. Resist the temptation to always have the last word and to always win an argument. Your marriage is more important that winning an argument and peace in your marriage is more profitable than have the last word.

Daily to do list

1) Read your why to each other.
2) Read the short daily devotional and meditate
3) Go out and exercise together
4) Focus on silence and what that means to you and your relationship. Challenge each other during your exercise on ways to incorporate silence in your marriage.
5) At the end of the day make a journal entry here on your observations and major takeaways.

_____

_____

_____

_____

_____

_____

_____

_____

_____

_____

_____

_____

Sunday: Speak

"The ultimate tragedy is not the oppression
and cruelty by the bad people but the silence
over that by the good people."
Martin Luther King, Jr.

While "silence is gold", not speaking when you are supposed to speak according to Martin Luther King Jr. it is "the ultimate tragedy." Most of the time many of us speak when we are supposed to be silent and are silent when we are supposed to speak. The result is the we miss the "gold" and bring tragedy upon ourselves. The reason we speak when we are not supposed to speak, especially when it has to do with us blaming and shaming others, is because it strokes our egos and make us feel superior to others. On the other hand, we do not speak when we are supposed to because we are afraid to pay the price of speaking up. We allow fear and selfishness to hold us back and prevent us from doing what is right. If you do not speak up for the sake of your marriage who will? Who do you think will care more about the well being of your marriage more than you? The answer is obvious. Nobody cares about your marriage more than you. Therefore, you have to do all within your power to speak live and not death to your marriage. Consider the following powerful verse from the book of proverbs;

"The tongue has the power of life and death,
and those who love it will eat its fruit."
Proverbs 18.21

Each time you open your mouth to say anything, it is an opportunity to speak life or death, peace or sorry. You are having an opportunity to build or tear down. Blessed is the couple who have figured out when to be silent and when to speak words of hope, life, peace, joy, comfort, encouragement, and love. This is not just going to happen; you will have to be intentional about it by training yourself om how to speak using the right words. The well-being and alternate fate of your marriage depends on it.

Daily to do list

1) Read your why to each other.
2) Read the short daily devotional and meditate
3) Take your weight and log it here: _____
4) Go out and exercise together
5) Focus on determination and what that means to you and your relationship. Challenge each other during your exercise on ways to incorporate determination in your marriage.
6) At the end of the day make a journal entry here on your observations and major takeaways.
7) Both of you have to compare notes, evaluate your progress, and make adjustments accordingly.

_____

_____

_____

_____

_____

_____

_____

_____

_____

Monday: Do

*"Better to do something imperfectly than
to do nothing perfectly."*
Robert H. Schuller

This has been an amazing journey and we are so proud of you for sticking to it. Today is a reminder of the power of doing. You are already a doer that is why for the past 63 days you are your wife or husband have religiously gone out to exercise. You are not only a hearer but a doer of what this whole journey has been about. When it comes to doing there are many different categories of people, those that want to do it perfectly, those that are waiting for the perfect conditions to do it and those that do not want to do it no matter what. We are not going to address each particular group because no matter how "good" your excuse is, if you do not do you will not get any results. This along should move you from a none doer to a doer. The benefits of doing are so great that you should do because you can only gain when you do. Perfection is not the goal, although it can be an exciting by product. Start by doing then all other things will fall into place, but do not allow the need to be perfect to prevent you from doing what you are supposed to do. It is in doing that we learn and grow. If we do not do there is no change and no results. All the ideas that we are are only ideas no matter how great they are. If we do not do what is required to achieve whatever is promised our goals dreams and aspirations are just wishful thoughts, because they will never see they light of day. Talk s cheap, but it is costly to do the right thing. The cost is not always monetary, it can be relationships, promotion, etc. How valuable is your marriage and how much are you willing to sacrifice for it to be great? You may have to let go the promotion opportunity or the next career move for the sake of your marriage. Maybe it is time to change your career so that the quality of your marriage can improve. Whatever you need to do now is the time to do it. So just do it!

Daily to do list

1) Read your why to each other.
2) Read the short daily devotional and meditate
3) Go out and exercise together
4) Focus on forgiveness and what that means to you and your relationship. Challenge each other during your exercise on ways to incorporate forgiveness in your marriage.
5) At the end of the day make a journal entry here on your observations and major takeaways.

_____

_____

_____

_____

_____

_____

_____

_____

_____

_____

_____

_____

_____

_____

Tuesday: Mistakes

*"A man must be big enough to admit his mistakes,
smart enough to profit from them, and strong
enough to correct them."*
John C. Maxwell

We all make mistakes and should be open about it. The problem is not in the mistake it is what we do after we make a mistake that matters the most. Many authors have suggested that instead of falling backwards you should fall forward. In other words, do not waste your mistakes, but learn from them. It does not matter how bad the mistake is, you must look for a way to heal and keep moving. Mistakes only become deadly if you stop moving, after you falter. But if you pick yourself up and march on you will benefit from the mistake.

My husband came home one day and was looking down casted and perplexed. After a while he told me that he had made a terrible and irreparable mistake and did not know what to do. For more than two weeks he had been preparing hard to give a keynote speech at a high school graduation. He was excited about the opportunity and told me earlier that morning that he was going to get his doctoral robe to wear the next day. Little did he know that the event was on Thursday and he had mistakenly assumed that the graduation was on Saturday. We are now on Friday and he is eagerly preparing to give a speech in an occasion that had already passed, and he was not aware. He found out when he was out of the house because he saw a missed message from the person who booked him to come speak, inquiring where he was. Shockingly for my husband the phone call was a day old. When he put one and one together the bitter truth hit him hard. He had missed the graduation ceremony and there was nothing he could do about it. But I was impressed how he handled it. On Monday he went to toastmasters and gave a speech about his mistake, encouraging his listeners to laugh at themselves when they make mistakes, share their experience with others and lean from their mistakes. He learned that scheduling appointments on a calendar is a smart thing to do.

Daily to do list

1) Read your why to each other.
2) Read the short daily devotional and meditate
3) Go out and exercise together
4) Focus on forgiveness and what that means to you and your relationship. Challenge each other during your exercise on ways to incorporate forgiveness in your marriage.
5) At the end of the day make a journal entry here on your observations and major takeaways.

_____

_____

_____

_____

_____

_____

_____

_____

_____

_____

Wednesday: Mother in-law

"My mother-in-law said, 'One day I will dance on your grave.'
I said 'I hope you do; I will be buried at sea."
Les Dawson

If you are married there are in-laws involved in your marriage or were involved at some point. To some couples the mentioning of in-laws especially mother in-laws send chills down their spines. There are too many horror mother in-law stories that we will never stop if we wanted to get into them. We do not have the time to get on the negative side of things because solutions are better than complaining. You must be aware of some of the root causes of mother in-law daughter in-law problems. The main culprits are jealousy, fear, and fear. The mother is afraid that her daughter in-law will not be able take proper care of her son. But she fails to understand that she was rising her son to leave someday and start his own family. It is not necessary for mother in-laws to be so fearful. Sons have always gotten married and will continue to do. It seems the mother in-laws forget that their won husbands were the sons also.

Some daughter in-laws are jealous of the love between more and son. They are afraid that their husband may not have enough love left for them if they love their mothers. This is sad, because the love a son has for his mother is love cannot be traded for the love he has for his wife. The tragedy arises when some foolish wives insist that their husbands have to choose between their mother and them. No wife should ever set their husband up for such an unnecessary drama. Dot not let fear and jealousy ruin your marriage.

Both the mother in-law and daughter in-law may convince themselves that they are doing it for the well-being of the son, husband, but it is out of selfishness, fear and jealousy and should be avoided at all cost both parties.

Daily to do list

1) Read your why to each other.
2) Read the short daily devotional and meditate
3) Go out and exercise together
4) Focus on forgiveness and what that means to you and your relationship. Challenge each other during your exercise on ways to incorporate forgiveness in your marriage.
5) At the end of the day make a journal entry here on your observations and major takeaways.

_____

_____

_____

_____

_____

_____

_____

_____

_____

_____

_____

_____

_____

Thursday: Father In-law

"I have a very successful father-in-law and family with very different political views."
Gavin Newsom

D o father in-laws bring in some of the tensions that mother in-laws bring in marriages? It depends on who you ask. But it seems most father in-laws just get along. But if fear is making some fasters too protective of their children or interfering in their marriages in a way that is not constructive this has to be discouraged. The goal of each parent should be to raise their children to someday leave the house and establish successful homes that are ran by them and not remote controlled and manipulated by their parents. When your children are young you have full control, but as they grow older you have to understand that they are developing their own mind and need some allowance to be themselves. It is unacceptable for parents to treat their adult children as if they were kindergarteners, by expecting them to consult them before taking any decision and on how to run and manage their homes.

No matter what happens it is not advisable to allow differing political views to separate families. The 2016 presidential elections in the United States of America brought President Trump to power and many democrats loathed and hated him to the point where friendships of decades were destroyed, and some families torn apart. Why? It is an election and at the end of the day another opportunity will come up for a different candidate to be elected, but your in-laws are going to be with you for a long time. Therefore, do not allow politics to ruin your relationships, especially with your in-laws.

Daily to do list

1) Read your why to each other.
2) Read the short daily devotional and meditate
3) Go out and exercise together
4) Focus on forgiveness and what that means to you and your relationship. Challenge each other during your exercise on ways to incorporate forgiveness in your marriage.
5) At the end of the day make a journal entry here on your observations and major takeaways.

_____

_____

_____

_____

_____

_____

_____

_____

_____

_____

_____

_____

_____

_____

_____

Friday: Children

"The most important thing a father can do
for his children is to love their mother."
Theodore Hesburgh

"Children are a blessing and the fruit of the union between a husband
and wife. In fact, the Psalmist says, "Children are a heritage from
the Lord, offspring a reward from him. Like arrows in the hands of
a warrior are children born in one's youth. Blessed is the man whose
quiver is full of them they will not be put to shame when
they contend with their opponents in court."
Psalms 127:3-5

B ut if couples are not careful this wonderful blessing of children can ruin their marriage. This can happen when the husband and wife neglect their relationship in order to take care of their children. There is nothing wrong in taking care of your children, but it should not be done at the expense of the marriage. The children will be with you for just a while and will leave you to go start their own families. After they leave you will be left with your husband or wife. Therefore, you better learn to get along with your husband or wife because you are going to be together for a long time.

Daily to do list

1) Read your why to each other.
2) Read the short daily devotional and meditate
3) Go out and exercise together
4) Focus on forgiveness and what that means to you and your relationship. Challenge each other during your exercise on ways to incorporate forgiveness in your marriage.
5) At the end of the day make a journal entry here on your observations and major takeaways.

_____

_____

_____

_____

_____

_____

_____

_____

_____

_____

_____

_____

_____

_____

_____

_____

_____

Day 69

Saturday: Pets

"I think people are obsessed with their pets because pets don't speak. It's that simple. After you hang up the phone, you never hear a dog say, 'You're a liar, and you are making the same self-sabotaging mistakes that have kept you single for far too long."
Taylor Negron

Pete was raised in a home with two dogs and throughout his life they always had a dog. As the years went by Pete developed a deep love an attachment to dogs and made up his mind that when he will always have a dog as a pet. Then he met Deborah in graduate school, and they fell in love and got married after graduation. During their courtship the discussed many things including the place pets were going to play in their lives, because Deborah was raised in a house without any pets and was not very fun of pets. That is why they decided that they will have just one dog when they moved in together and Pete will be careful not to spend too much time with the dog.

After they got married Pete did all to spend time with Deborah, but slowly started spending more time with their golden retriever. The issue was that Pete was working too hard and coming home late, the least amount of time he had, he had to divide it between his wife, their daughter and their dog and it seems the dog was wining. Deborah was too busy taking care of their baby that she had no time to take the dog out for a walk. And did not care very much for it because it was something she did not enjoy doing.

Pete will comeback from work and all he though was taking the dog out for a walk. When asked why he was giving preference to the dog over his daughter Pete was of the opinion that his wife was spending enough time with their daughter already, but their dog was being neglected. Their marriage was being threatened because of the pet, yet none of them was willing to compromise. The more the insisted on having their way, the deeper the right between them widened.

Daily to do list

1) Read your why to each other.
2) Read the short daily devotional and meditate
3) Go out and exercise together
4) Focus on your pets and what that means to you and your relationship. Challenge each other during your exercise on ways your pets may be impacting your marriage.
5) At the end of the day make a journal entry here on your observations and major takeaways.

_____

_____

_____

_____

_____

_____

_____

_____

_____

_____

_____

_____

Sunday: Old Friends

"Remember that the most valuable
antiques are dear old friends."
H. Jackson Brown, Jr.

Abu was known as "the man of the people" by his friends before he met Fatima. Theirs was love at first sight and they were soon married, and it was not long after that Fatima's true colors began to manifest. During the short period of their courtship Fatima had given the impression that she enjoyed having company over and meeting new people. In fact, she had attended all the parties that Abu had been invited to. She went along with the long list of invitees Abu put together for their wedding. The wedding was greatly attended and high successful. Abu's friends could not let him down because he had been there for them as well.

But things changed after they got married. Initially Abu thought Fatima was just adjusting to her new environment and role as his wife, because she started feeling reluctant to accept invitations for both of them to go out and for people to come over and visit. She always came up with one complain or the other. The few times they went out she will not have anything good to say about the friends they had spent the evening with. When Abu's friends came over to visit, she did not put up a good face and Abu's friends started withdrawing from him and not too long none of his friends would come over to visit him, nor will they invite him for their functions. In short Abu's old friendships were ruined not too long after he got married. Although this did not sit well with him, he was helpless on what to do.

Avoid destroying your old friendships because they are extremely valuable.

Daily to do list

1) Read your why to each other.
2) Read the short daily devotional and meditate
3) Take your weight and log it here_____
4) Go out and exercise together
5) Focus on determination and what that means to you and your relationship. Challenge each other during your exercise on ways to incorporate determination in your marriage.
6) At the end of the day make a journal entry here on your observations and major takeaways.
7) Both of you have to compare notes, evaluate your progress and make adjustments accordingly.

_____

_____

_____

_____

_____

_____

_____

_____

_____

_____

_____

Monday: Relationships

"When we understand the connection between how we live and how long we live, it's easier to make different choices. Instead of viewing the time we spend with friends and family as luxuries, we can see that these relationships are among the most powerful determinants of our well-being and survival."
Dean Ornish

We were created for relationships, because of that the quality of our relationships influence the quality of our lives. Therefore, it is imperative for each husband and wife to nurture their marriage and in addition to that the other relationships in their lives have to be created for as well. Do not be a loner, because you need other people especially your extended family. Some husbands and wives make the mistake of cut everybody off and when they hit a hard patch do not have any body to turn to. You and your husband or wife should do all to resolve your differences and difficulties that may come your way. But at times you may need a second opinion and it is important that you have people who know you well enough that they can make a meaningful contribution in your life. When all is going well with you, there is the tendency to feel that you are invincible and need nobody, until disaster hits and you realize that you are vulnerable and need the love and support of other people.

Life is more enjoyable, fulfilling and satisfying when it is shared with others. There is a great temptation to try and be a lone ranger, resist it by cultivating and nurturing other relationships, for you are going need them.

Daily to do list

1) Read your why to each other.
2) Read the short daily devotional and meditate
3) Go out and exercise together
4) Focus on forgiveness and what that means to you and your relationship. Challenge each other during your exercise on ways to incorporate forgiveness in your marriage.
5) At the end of the day make a journal entry here on your observations and major takeaways.

_____

_____

_____

_____

_____

_____

_____

_____

_____

_____

_____

_____

_____

_____

_____

_____

_____

Tuesday: Mental Toughness

*"Mental toughness is Spartacism with
qualities of sacrifice, self-denial, dedication.
It is fearlessness, and it is love."*
Vince Lombardi

Why do some succeed, and others fail? This question can be asked about marriages as well. If you look around you will realize that some of the couples that got married at the same time with you are no longer married. If you have been paying attention as well, you must have noticed that a week does not pass without you hearing about a marriage that has fallen apart or running into somebody that has divorced. What is going on? Why do people start with such excitement and end up bitter and disappointed? What can be done to prevent this from happening? Is your own marriage immune to it falling apart? Do you have what it takes to make it to the end?

These questions are not being asked to put anybody on the spotlight, but it is for us to ponder and look for solutions. The pain that is associated with failed marriages and eventually divorce is nothing something that anybody wants to or should go through. All has to be done to mitigate and even prevent marriages from failing. We wrote this manual and the book that accompanies it, because we want to bring solutions to the table. Our hope is that marriages will be strengthened, and sick ones healed.

One secret to having a divorced proof marriage is developing mental toughness, as the Legendary Dallas Cowboys Football coach Vince Lombardi puts it, "Mental toughness is Spartacism with qualities of sacrifice, self-denial, dedication. It is fearlessness, and it is love." You have to make up your mind and be committed to the promises you have made to each other and stick to your guns no matter what. Exercising together will help your development and give you some mental toughness as well. We are glad you have taken this 90-day challenge seriously.

Daily to do list

1) Read your why to each other.
2) Read the short daily devotional and meditate
3) Go out and exercise together
4) Focus on forgiveness and what that means to you and your relationship. Challenge each other during your exercise on ways to incorporate forgiveness in your marriage.
5) At the end of the day make a journal entry here on your observations and major takeaways.

_____

_____

_____

_____

_____

_____

_____

_____

_____

_____

Wednesday: Vision

*"I've learned that fear limits you and your vision. It serves as blinders
to what may be just a few steps down the road for you. The journey
is valuable, but believing in your talents, your abilities, and your
self-worth can empower you to walk down an even brighter path.
Transforming fear into freedom – how great is that?"*
Soledad O'Brien

Each time you hear of vision what come into your mind? Do you think of some supernatural and miraculous encounter with angles? We are going to be using vision in this context to refer to what you are "seeing" regarding your marriage. This "seeing" has nothing to do with the physical eyes, but everything to do with your spiritual eyes. Do you see you and your husband or wife getting old together and staying married until death parts you? Do you see both of you have an exciting fun filled marriage? Do you see your romantic life blossoming and both of you enjoying each other's company? Do you see you and your husband or wife having less arguments and fighting? Do you see your marriage growing stronger with each passing day?

What you see will determine what you believe and what you believe will influence your actions. The outcome of your life is directly proportional to your actions. When you align your thoughts, beliefs, and actions you will achieve what you are seeing. If all you see is failure and separation, it will be unto you according to your measure of faith. Those see failure, separation, and divorce as the ultimate fate of their marriage act accordingly. They do not pay attention to nurturing the marriage and will not be reading a manual like this. But we hope that your case is different, and you truly see and few in your marriage, that is why you are on this journey. The vison for your marriage is not something supernatural. You made a vow to love, cherish and be with each other till death parts you. This is the covenant that was agreed upon and you should see yourself sticking to the end. When you make up your mind concerning this all other things will follow.

Daily to do list

1) Read your why to each other.
2) Read the short daily devotional and meditate
3) Go out and exercise together
4) Focus on vison and what that means to you and your relationship. Challenge each other during your exercise on ways to incorporate vison in your marriage.
5) At the end of the day make a journal entry here on your observations and major takeaways.

_____

_____

_____

_____

_____

_____

_____

_____

_____

_____

_____

_____

Thursday: Belief

"Our beliefs create the kind of world we believe in. We project our feelings, thoughts and attitudes onto the world. I can create a different world by changing my belief about the world. Our inner state creates the outer and not vice versa."
John Bradshaw

Belief is so important that our physical reality is control by our belief system. Take for example those who believe that an airplane is unsafe are said to have a phobia for flying. Some of these individuals has such a strong phobia that they never fly at all. There are many other phobias that people have, and it prevents them from traveling, eating, and doing many things that many of us take for granted. What started in their minds is not having physical manifestation with serious ramifications.

Your marriage is not immune to your beliefs, and they will make or break your marriage. Therefore, any husband and wife that need a strong, robust, and lasting marriage must take the belief system seriously. The dangers of believing in the wrong way are real and should not be taken lightly by any married couple. If you believe that your marriage will fail, or that it is no good and there is no point investing in it, the marriage will suffer neglect and will implode eventually. Here are some powerful Bible verses that will help you tremendously;

"Finally, brothers and sisters, whatever is true, whatever is noble, whatever is right, whatever is pure, whatever is lovely, whatever is admirable—if anything is excellent or praiseworthy—think about such things. Whatever you have learned or received or heard from me or seen in me—put it into practice. And the God of peace will be with you."
Philippians 4:8-9 New International Version (NIV)

Memorize these verses and used them to defeat those beliefs that are contrary to the wellbeing of your marriage, your health and your life and you will walk in victory.

Daily to do list

1) Read your why to each other.
2) Read the short daily devotional and meditate
3) Go out and exercise together
4) Focus on forgiveness and what that means to you and your relationship. Challenge each other during your exercise on ways to incorporate forgiveness in your marriage.
5) At the end of the day make a journal entry here on your observations and major takeaways.

_____

_____

_____

_____

_____

_____

_____

_____

_____

_____

Friday: Anxiety

"The truth is that there is no actual stress or anxiety in the world; it's your thoughts that create these false beliefs. You can't package stress, touch it, or see it. There are only people engaged in stressful thinking."
Wayne Dyer

Are you giving life to the monsters that are hunting you? It is possible to turn an anthill into an insurmountable mountain if you focus intensely on the anthill. If you want to try the power of focus take a penny close one of your eyes with one hand, use the other hand to hold the penny in front of the open eye. The next thing is to slowly bring the penny close to your eye. You will realize that the closer you bring the penny to your eye the bigger the penny will get because it begins to shield everything else. You will eventually not able to see anything else because your focus is the penny and nothing else. But if you remove the penny and compare it to the world around you, the penny will pale into comparison to other things in the room or around you. Are you turning the little pennies in your life into mountains? Anxiety, and panic attacks are a result of focusing intensely on your problems or challenges that are surrounding you. The best thing to do is focus on the possibilities and solutions because there is always a way out.

Dealing with anxiety requires mental toughness and you will need a lot of help to do that. We are suggesting that you use the following tried and proven approach to defeat anxiety when it shows its ugly head and threaten to destroy your life and your marriage.

"Do not be anxious about anything, but in every situation, by prayer and petition, with thanksgiving, present your requests to God. And the peace of God, which transcends all understanding, will guard your hearts and your minds in Christ Jesus." Philippians 4 New International Version (NIV)

Daily to do list

1) Read your why to each other.
2) Read the short daily devotional and meditate
3) Go out and exercise together
4) Focus on forgiveness and what that means to you and your relationship. Challenge each other during your exercise on ways to incorporate forgiveness in your marriage.
5) At the end of the day make a journal entry here on your observations and major takeaways.

_____

_____

_____

_____

_____

_____

_____

_____

_____

_____

_____

_____

_____

Day 76

Saturday: Assumption

"I can't say that the ending of a story is always the best part of the story, and yet there's sort of this implicit idea that the finale is somehow supposed to be the mind-blowing best episode of a show. The question is: Why is that? Why do people make that assumption?"
Carlton Cuse

What are some of the assumptions that have landed you into trouble? Because you made some assumptions you draw conclusions and took certain decisions that led to disastrous actions. One pillar stone to proper communication is to avoid making assumptions. You must make sure that you have as much information as possible and all the data that you can gather before making any conclusions. A failure to let the data lead you can lead to a disaster in your marriage. Just because something appears to be good or bad does not meant that it is. It is your responsibility to test every spirit and to make sure that things add up before you take any action. If in doubt, ask and keep on asking until you get the answer that you need. Nobody says this better than James the Apostle,

My dear brothers and sisters, take note of this: Everyone should be quick to listen, slow to speak and slow to become angry, because human anger does not produce the righteousness that God desires. James 1:19 New International Version (NIV)

This is such a powerful, commonsense and life changing reminder to all husbands and wives to be "be quick to listen, slow to speak and slow to become angry." Any husband and wife that take this admonition at heart and actually apply it will save themselves from a lot of unnecessary pain and heartache. It takes effort to listen and a lot of restraint not to speak all what is in your mind.

Daily to do list

1) Read your why to each other.
2) Read the short daily devotional and meditate
3) Go out and exercise together
4) Focus on forgiveness and what that means to you and your relationship. Challenge each other during your exercise on ways to incorporate forgiveness in your marriage.
5) At the end of the day make a journal entry here on your observations and major takeaways.

_____

_____

_____

_____

_____

_____

_____

_____

_____

_____

_____

_____

_____

_____

_____

_____

Day 77

Sunday: Intentional

"You don't climb mountains without a team, you don't climb mountains without being fit, you don't climb mountains without being prepared and you don't climb mountains without balancing the risks and rewards. And you never climb a mountain on accident – it has to be intentional."
Mark Udall

Joe and Monique found themselves in the office of a marriage counselor one cold and snowy morning in January, then it hit them that there were in deep trouble. Their marriage was falling apart, and they felt helpless on what to do. Part of their shock was the fact that they had vowed to each other that they will never allow themselves to get to the point where the services of a counsellor will be required and that they will always be there for each other, love support and do whatever it takes to ensure that their marriage was strong, exciting and rewarding.

Both of them had meet on a mission trip to Honduras and discovered that they shared a lot in common and had similar goals and aspiration. After they got married, they prayed together every morning, attend church regularly and told each other "I love you" at the end of each day. Their marriage was a beacon of light to many and other couples came to them for advice and encouragement. Then something changed. It was not a sudden change and did not appear to be anything major. Joe got a promotion at work and the work demand kept increasing and he started getting up very early to go to work. They had bought a bigger house and needed the money to keep up with payments. In addition to the change in Joe's job situation, they had twin babies. Initially their plan was for Monique to stay at home and look after the babies, but she had to keep working because in addition to the new house, they were having a boat and a beach house to pay for. All these pressures caused them to gradually stop doing those little things that made their marriage great and not too longer they were constantly on each other's throat.

Daily to do list

1) Read your why to each other.
2) Read the short daily devotional and meditate
3) Take your weight and log it here: _____
4) Go out and exercise together
5) Focus on intentionality and what that means to you and your relationship. Challenge each other during your exercise on ways to incorporate intentionality in your marriage.
6) At the end of the day make a journal entry here on your observations and major takeaways.
7) Both of you have to compare notes, evaluate your progress, and make adjustments accordingly.

_____

_____

_____

_____

_____

_____

_____

_____

_____

_____

Monday: Proactive

"To be a proactive person, you must learn to say no to most ideas and opportunities, so you have the mental and physical bandwidth to execute the realistic business plans you have already mapped out."
Clay Clark

If you do not have a battle plan, it is will be disastrous to try and come up with one in the heat of battle. Having a battle plan before the battle is an indication that you are proactive. You are anticipating what is going to happened and making preparation for it. Unfortunately, many husbands and wives wait for disaster to hit before they scramble to figure out what to do to get out.

When Anna and Paul got married the decided that they were never going to allow a job to separate them, because they were prioritizing their marriage. In addition to this decision they also promised each other that immediate their first child arrived Anna will stay at home and take care of the child. After three years of marriage, Anna became pregnant and when she gave birth she had to resign from her position as the gynecologist in one of the Methodists hospitals in her city. Paul was the manger in one of the telecom companies in their city and was doing well. But a few days after Anna resigned her job, the dot com burst happened, and Paul was laid off. They moved from a two-income family to a zero-income family within a matter of days. Fortunately for them they had about an emergency fund that was able to pay for their expenses over a five-month period. The severance package that Paul got when he was laid off also helped some.

Paul started looking for work immediately, but there were none and after six months with their emergency fund running out, Paul got a call from an out of town recruiter from a major Telcom company that needed is expertise badly, but the job required a lot of traveling in and out of the country. Paul and Anna thought about it and decided that Paul should turn down the offer.

Daily to do list

1) Read your why to each other.
2) Read the short daily devotional and meditate
3) Go out and exercise together
4) Focus on forgiveness and what that means to you and your relationship. Challenge each other during your exercise on ways to incorporate forgiveness in your marriage.
5) At the end of the day make a journal entry here on your observations and major takeaways.

_____

_____

_____

_____

_____

_____

_____

_____

_____

_____

_____

_____

_____

Tuesday: Temptation

"For years my wedding ring has done its job. It has led me not into temptation. It has reminded my husband numerous times at parties that it's time to go home. It has been a source of relief to a dinner companion. It has been a status symbol in the maternity ward."
Erma Bombeck

If you are living on this earth you will be tempted sooner or later, but you can overcome the temptation as well. Take the case of Lisa who is highly qualified and has been doing a good job at work, but her boss keeps passing her when promotion times comes. One time on a busy trip her boss called her to come up in his hotel room during a launch break and when she got in, he tried to have sex with her under the condition that she will get promoted and make more money. The offer was tempting, because she was going to able to afford some of the things right up to that moment she had only dreamt of. But she was married and there was no way she was going to break her marriage vow. The boss pulled out the drafted letter and all the benefits and pleaded with her that it was a onetime something and nobody will ever know about it therefore she should not be worried about being caught or exposed. Lisa was not going to have any of it and stormed out of the room. His boss was notorious for using his position of power and influence to have his way with women, married and unmarried. Nobody in the company had the courage to confront him, because he was the son-in-law of the owner of the company. Secondly in the county were Lisa lived, it was commonplace for bosses to take advantage of women because of weak laws against such practices and little or no enforcement.

Unfortunately for Lisa's boss, Lisa understood and believed what this Bible verse teaches.

"No temptation[s] has overtaken you except what is common to mankind. And God is faithful; he will not let you be tempted beyond what you can bear. But when you are tempted, he will also provide a way out so that you can endure it." 1 Corinthians 10:13 New International Version (NIV)

We are human and get tempted, but no temptation is more than and here is always a way out of it.

Daily to do list

1) Read your why to each other.
2) Read the short daily devotional and meditate
3) Go out and exercise together
4) Focus on forgiveness and what that means to you and your relationship. Challenge each other during your exercise on ways to incorporate forgiveness in your marriage.
5) At the end of the day make a journal entry here on your observations and major takeaways.

_____

_____

_____

_____

_____

_____

_____

_____

_____

_____

Day 80

Wednesday: Endurance

"Endurance training is so mental. You just do it. You just can, and you just will, and you just run that far because, you know, I get tired at the first mile. I feel heavy and all of those things, but now I have developed, it's hard to explain... It's a very satisfying place to get into."
Paul Sparks

One of the secretes of all successful and enduring marriages is endurance. The husband and wife must develop thick skin, dig in their heels and "just do it." They do not allow what is popular to lead them, nor do they try to be like the everybody. The husband and wife understand that, just because it is popular does not mean that it is right and also, they know feelings can be misleading at times. This husband and wife team understand that anything worth having is worth fighting for. They accept the fact that any good marriage needs a lot of hard work, time, and energy.

Each day they motivate themselves to keep working and investing in their marriage. You often find them at the end of the day counting their blessings and reminding each other of past victories, failures, and good times. They are not afraid to plan their future and work towards it, because they belief in each other and in their marriage and are willing to pay the price to walk the talk. Their marriage is not just an afterthought, but it is at the center of who they are and what they do.

Take the case of Amina and Hans, they come from a culture where having children is highly priced and those who are married but do have children become the talk of the community. It is not uncommon for childless marriages to implode because of pressures from the family of the husband. This is why after 12 years of marriage and no child, Amina and Hans were under immense pressure to do something because Hans's parents were insisting that he sends away and get married to a different woman who would bare them grandchildren. Hans was not having any of it and refused to send Amina away. After 15 enduring years, Amina became pregnant.

Daily to do list

1) Read your why to each other.
2) Read the short daily devotional and meditate
3) Go out and exercise together
4) Focus on forgiveness and what that means to you and your relationship. Challenge each other during your exercise on ways to incorporate forgiveness in your marriage.
5) At the end of the day make a journal entry here on your observations and major takeaways.

_____

_____

_____

_____

_____

_____

_____

_____

_____

_____

Thursday: Pressure

"I just feel like, with growing up and having peer pressure and what society wants you to be and what you think you should do, I feel like it's really important to surround yourself around good, understanding, amazing people that actually love you for you."
Storm Reid

Daily to do list

1) Read your why to each other.
2) Read the short daily devotional and meditate
3) Go out and exercise together
4) Focus on forgiveness and what that means to you and your relationship. Challenge each other during your exercise on ways to incorporate forgiveness in your marriage.
5) At the end of the day make a journal entry here on your observations and major takeaways.

Friday: Conformity

"So many people live within unhappy circumstances and yet will not take the initiative to change their situation because they are conditioned to a life of security, conformity, and conservation, all of which may appear to give one peace of mind, but in reality, nothing is more damaging to the adventurous spirit."
Christopher McCandless

Just because everybody else is doing it, does not mean that you should do it. Your marriage is not just any other marriage, because you are your wife or husband are unique. This implies that your marriage is unique, and you must see your marriage in that light. If you fail to understand and celebrate your uniqueness you will end up like everybody else, but you are not everybody else, you are different, and it is Okay to be different.

Conformity leads to group thinking and group thinking is dangerous. By default, humans like what is familiar, predictable, and comfortable, even when it is not to their full advantage. The need to belong and be part of a group trumps everything for most people and they end up conforming instead of transforming their environment and circumstances. The process of transforming your circumstances and reinventing yourself starts with the refusal to conform. Here is what Paul the apostil says concerning transformation and growth;

"Do not conform to the pattern of this world but be transformed by the renewing of your mind. Then you will be able to test and approve what God's will is—his good, pleasing and perfect will." Romans 12:2 New International Version (NIV)

Your marriage is different from other marriages and you should not be ashamed to affirm and maintain the uniqueness of your marriage. Your goal should be to look like everyone else or to fit it. Let your goal be focused on being all God created you and brought you and your husband or wife together to be. Resist the temptation and pressure from society to conform!

Daily to do list

1) Read your why to each other.
2) Read the short daily devotional and meditate
3) Go out and exercise together
4) Focus on forgiveness and what that means to you and your relationship. Challenge each other during your exercise on ways to incorporate forgiveness in your marriage.
5) At the end of the day make a journal entry here on your observations and major takeaways.

_____

_____

_____

_____

_____

_____

_____

_____

_____

_____

Day 83

Saturday: Opposition

"Just as we develop our physical muscles through overcoming opposition – such as lifting weights – we develop our character muscles by overcoming challenges and adversity."
Stephen Covey

You are going to be opposed if you not already been. We this because many people want you to be like them and when they see you making progress towards your goals, they will not like it. Do not be surprised when your friends start telling you that exercising regularly with your wife or husband is not such a great idea. They will even accuse you of showing off when you share with them what you are doing. Why will those who you think should be cheering you on and encouraging you to take care of your health and strengthen your marriage oppose you? The answer lies in the fact that when you are doing something people know they are supposed to be doing but are not doing they hate it. The hatred from those who are not doing what you are doing is based on the fact that you are reminding them that it is possible to do what they have been procrastinating or have said it is impossible to do. In some cases when you are succeeding those who tried and failed are reminded of their own failure and this robs them babdly. Instead of them using your success as inspiration to try again, they turn their frustration and defeat to hate. Unfortunately, some of these people are unconsciously opposing without processing it.

Therefore, when you are opposed you should not overreact, because those opposing you may not be aware of what they are doing. The best approach is to keep calm and keep going. If these individuals become verbally abuses, it may be time to give some gap between you and them. Opposition is not a bad thing; it is how you respond to it that will determine the outcome that you get. If you see opposition as an opportunity to grow and develop metal toughness you will plough through it successfully.

Daily to do list

1) Read your why to each other.
2) Read the short daily devotional and meditate
3) Go out and exercise together
4) Focus on forgiveness and what that means to you and your relationship. Challenge each other during your exercise on ways to incorporate forgiveness in your marriage.
5) At the end of the day make a journal entry here on your observations and major takeaways.

_____

_____

_____

_____

_____

_____

_____

_____

_____

_____

_____

_____

_____

Sunday: Doubt

"I remember my choir teacher in high school told me, 'When in doubt, sing loud.' I'm a terrible singer, but I always auditioned for the musicals, and would get cast in them because I really would just put it all out there." That was really good advice, and I think it works for everything, not just acting."
Judy Greer

You are married to the right people and should stop doubting if you made the right decision or not. Doubt is fueled by fear, especially the failure of failure of losing something that you hold dear or desire to have. Therefore, do not allow fear to destroy your marriage. If you ask all those who have been married for many years and their marriages are doing well, they will tell you that commitment is the chief cornerstone of their marriage. They do not get up each morning and check their feelings towards each other. This is not to say that feelings are not important in marriage. Feelings have their place, but any marriage that is based on feelings or allows feelings to lead the way will end up in a ditch.

This is why all successful marriages are led by commitment, the husbands and wives in this marriage have learned over the years that, feelings come and go, but commitment is a solid rock. When the get up each they, their focus is not how they are feeling, but on the promise, they made to love, hold, and cherish their husband or wife under all circumstances. This implies that the conditions surrounding them do not determine the outcome of their marriage but commitment overrides everything. Therefore, when in doubt if you are still in love with your husband or wife you should remember that you made a commitment to love them no matter what. You are not the only person battling doubt, but it only wins when you forget out promise to each other.

Daily to do list

1) Read your why to each other.
2) Read the short daily devotional and meditate
3) Take your weight and log it here: _____
4) Go out and exercise together
5) Focus on doubt and what that means to you and your relationship. Challenge each other during your exercise on ways to get rid of doubt from your marriage.
6) At the end of the day make a journal entry here on your observations and major takeaways.
7) Both of you have to compare notes, evaluate your progress and make adjustments accordingly.

_____

_____

_____

_____

_____

_____

_____

_____

_____

_____

_____

Monday: Disappointment

"Our heavenly Father understands our disappointment, suffering, pain, fear, and doubt. He is always there to encourage our hearts and help us understand that He's sufficient for all of our needs. When I accepted this as an absolute truth in my life, I found that my worrying stopped."
Charles Stanley

Have you been disappointed? May be not as many times as Ashu who got engaged to his high school sweetheart and on the day of their weeding his fiancée was killed in an accident on her way to the church for the weeding. The marriage convey was descending a hill when the brakes of an eighteen-wheeler failed, and it crushed the limousine Ashu's fiancé was riding in. It was not long after this sad and disappointing incident that Ashu's warehouse caught fire and was completely burned down destroying everything in it. Many people suggested that he should leave the city and move somewhere else because some of his close friends abandoned him and will not call or pick up his calls. What made it even more painful and extremely disappointing was the fact that some of these friends were doing well because Ashu had not only mentored them, he had provided them with the capital to start their own businesses.

You might not have been through anything as traumatic as Ashu but have had your own share of disappointments and these may be threatening to undue your marriage because each time you try to move forward the disappointment tries to hold you back. The trust you had for one another has been eroded and you are finding it had to trust. Some of the high hopes and expectations you had for each other has been dashed and now you are disappointed and may even be considering getting out of the relationship. We suggest not so fast, there is hope and your Heavenly Father understands your pain, disappointment, and frustration. The best thing to do is to hand over all the pain, disappointment and frustration to him and He will take care of it for you.

Daily to do list

1) Read your why to each other.
2) Read the short daily devotional and meditate
3) Go out and exercise together
4) Focus on disappointments and what that means to you and your relationship. Challenge each other during your exercise on ways to limit the negative effects of disappointment on your marriage.
5) At the end of the day make a journal entry here on your observations and major takeaways.

_____

_____

_____

_____

_____

_____

_____

_____

_____

_____

_____

Thursday: Distractions

"Successful people maintain a positive focus in life no matter what is going on around them. They stay focused on their past successes rather than their past failures, and on the next action steps they need to take to get them closer to the fulfillment of their goals rather than all the other distractions that life presents to them."
Jack Canfield

There is so much against the marriage institution that each husband and wife have to on their guard at all times, because taking any chances is disastrous. The demands of modern living, the decline of the institution of marriage and the high divorce rate and push by some to redefine marriage are putting tremendous pressure on marriages. When you hear of people who have been married for more than 30 years divorcing, you must remind yourself that no marriage is immune including yours. There are too many distractions that are bent on destroying your marriage and these forces work 24/7, you too must up your game and stand firm against distractions.

Here is an admonition from the songs of Songs on what to do concerning the little foxes, "Catch for us the foxes, the little foxes that ruin the vineyards, our vineyards that are in bloom." Song of Songs 2:15 New International Version (NIV)

The instruction is simple, you have to catch all the little foxes that are ruining your marriage. Get rid of the people in your life that are advising you to be unfaithful to your mate, those that want you to walk in anger and resentment. Stop watching pornography, lusting, and flirting with other people. Cut back on the hours that you work and spend some quality time with your mate. You know what these little foxes are and now is the time to catch and destroy them before they ruin your marriage.

Daily to do list

1) Read your why to each other.
2) Read the short daily devotional and meditate
3) Go out and exercise together
4) Focus on the little foxes and what that means to you and your marriage. Challenge each other during your exercise on ways to get rid of all the little foxes in your marriage.
5) At the end of the day make a journal entry here on your observations and major takeaways.

_____

_____

_____

_____

_____

_____

_____

_____

_____

_____

_____

_____

_____

Monday: Hurt

"Hurt leads to bitterness, bitterness to anger, travel
too far that road and the way is lost."
Terry Brooks

If you are married and human, chances are you have been hurt and have hurt others. We are looking at hurt within the context of your marriage. As Bob Marley puts it, *"Truth is everybody is going to hurt you: you just gotta find the ones worth suffering for."* In other words you are going to be hurt and what will you do about it will determine the outcome that you get. Forgiveness as we have already discussed is the logical thing to do but it is easier said than done, because hurt breeds bitterness and if the bitterness is not starved it will lead to anger and resentment. If you continue on the path of anger and resentment you will do something stupid. The sooner you stop this madness the better. It is easier to forgive and love when you have experienced true unconditional love and forgiveness. This type of unconditional love and forgiveness is Divine love and the only place to go get it is getting connect to God. At the end of this manual we are going to show you how you can do that. And if you are not yet connected to God, you should seize the opportunity.

Mother Theresia adds another dimension to how the negative power of hurt can be harnessed to do good. She says that, *"I have found the paradox, that if you love until it hurts, there can be no more hurt, only more love." Keep loving is the solution that will take hurt out of business."* Here, mother Theresia is talking about the practically of dealing with hurt through love, because initially you will not like to, because it hurts, but if you persist the hurt will be completely displaced by love. She was not making this up, because the Bible already says that

"Above all, love each other deeply, because love covers over a multitude of sins." 1 Peter 4:8 New International Version (NIV)

Daily to do list

1) Read your why to each other.
2) Read the short daily devotional and meditate
3) Go out and exercise together
4) Focus on forgiveness and what that means to you and your relationship. Challenge each other during your exercise on ways to incorporate forgiveness in your marriage.
5) At the end of the day make a journal entry here on your observations and major takeaways.

_____

_____

_____

_____

_____

_____

_____

_____

_____

_____

_____

_____

_____

_____

Monday: Submission

"The success of the suffrage movement would injure women spiritually and intellectually, for they would be assuming a burden though they knew themselves unable to bear it. It is the sediment, not the wave, of a sex. It is the antithesis of that highest and sweetest mystery - conviction by submission, and conquest by sacrifice."
John Boyle O'Reilly

The subject of submission is a hot potato and we are not afraid to pick it. There is no way a strong and lasting marriage can be built without proper understanding of submission. There are extensive works on these subjects, and you should do your homework and explore it. Because failure to have a proper understanding and application of submission in the marriage will lead to disaster. Many people have falsely interpreted the call for submission to mean wife battery, demeaning and abuse. This is a far cry from what God intended. According to the following instructions it is a beautiful picture of sacrifice, love, harmony, and synergy, *"Submit to one another out of reverence for Christ."* Ephesians 5:21

Submission is not a one-way street, both husband and wife out of their free volition place themselves under each other. This has nothing to do with superiority, both husband and wife and equal, but their roles are different, this does not mean that any of the roles is better than the other.

Below is one of the verses that many feminists want to erase out of the Bible, because it says;

"Wives, submit yourselves to your own husbands as you do to the Lord. For the husband is the head of the wife as Christ is the head of the church, his body, of which he is the Savior. Now as the church submits to Christ, so also wives should submit to their husbands in everything."
Ephesians 5:22-24

If you meet any creature with two heads, you know it is not normal. When the woman is asked to submit to her husband because he is the head, it is for functionality and not positional. A body cannot function without the head and the head cannot do anything on its own. The head is nothing without the body. The husband being the head does not mean that he is superior to his wife. If you are a student of the Bible you will know that we are all one in Christ and there is no male or female, Jew or Gentile free or slave.

Some people think that the husband got a better deal, the truth is far from this. What the husband is charged with doing is serious and if all husbands are doing that, any woman in their right mind will willingly submit to them. All of us submit to Christ because of what He has done for us. Jesus sacrificed His life for our redemption. Husbands are being called to love their wives like Christ loved the church, here is how Paul the apostle puts it;

"Husbands, love your wives, just as Christ loved the church and gave himself up for her to make her holy, cleansing her by the washing with water through the word, and to present her to himself as a radiant church, without stain or wrinkle or any other blemish, but holy and blameless. In this same way, husbands ought to love their wives as their own bodies. He who loves his wife loves himself. After all, no one ever hated their own body, but they feed and care for their body, just as Christ does the church—for we are members of his body.

*"For this reason a man will leave his father and mother and be united
to his wife, and the two will become one flesh." This is a profound
mystery—but I am talking about Christ and the church. However, each
one of you also must love his wife as he loves himself, and the
wife must respect her husband."*
Ephesians 5:21

The husband is expected to love his wife just as he loves his own
body. Nobody in their right mind abuses, neglect and mistreats their
body. Therefore, any husband who is cruel to their wife and does not
treat them well is not living in obedience and should repent.

Submission will only work when the husband is doing what he
has been charged to do, and that is to love unconditionally. This is
extremely difficult and humanly impossible, that is why many fail at
it. The good news is that God's love is freely available to all who ask
for it. The ball starts with the husband and when they love their wives
as Christ loved the church, they will their wives will respect them
and be submissive to them. Love is more powerful than anything
else, therefore let the husbands strive to love. The wives have to be
respectful not out of fear but reverence that will make their husband
excel in and out of their home. It is a win, win for everybody. Never
forget that the wife is her husband's help mate and to help you must
be strong.

Daily to do list

1) Read your why to each other.
2) Read the short daily devotional and meditate
3) Go out and exercise together
4) Focus on forgiveness and what that means to you and your
   relationship. Challenge each other during your exercise on
   ways to incorporate forgiveness in your marriage.

5) At the end of the day make a journal entry here on your observations and major takeaways.

_____

_____

_____

_____

_____

_____

_____

_____

_____

_____

_____

_____

_____

_____

_____

_____

_____

_____

_____

_____

_____

Monday: Legacy

*"The greatest legacy one can pass on to one's children
and grandchildren is not money or other material
things accumulated in one's life, but rather a
legacy of character and faith."*
Billy Graham

Live does not end when you die. Therefore, you have to be considerate of the actions you take on a daily basis. If today was the last day of your life, how will you want to be remembered? Will today be the day you will want to represent you? If your answer is no, then you have a lot to do. Do you know that your life is going to be the sum of each single day? It is imperative that we understand that each day is an opportunity to sow good or bad seeds, to increase or decrease. Your legacy is being fashioned daily therefore each day matters a lot.

One crucial way your legacy will be measured is not the number of houses you built, the number of cars you had or promotions at work, it is going to be how well your children do. Here is an excellent definition of legacy through the lenses of your children and nobody does a better job than Naveen Jain who says,

*"I believe our legacy will be defined by the accomplishments and fearless
nature by which our daughters and sons take on the global challenges
we face. I also wonder if perhaps the most lasting expression of one's
humility lies in our ability to foster and mentor our children."*

This is not in any way suggesting that you are going to control the behavior of your children or be held responsible of their actions. But children do what they see and not what they are told. Your children will reflect what you are doing. That is why the best thing any father can do for his daughters is to unconditionally love their mother. When time comes your daughters will find a man like you.

Daily to do list

1) Read your why to each other.
2) Read the short daily devotional and meditate
3) Go out and exercise together
4) Focus on forgiveness and what that means to you and your relationship. Challenge each other during your exercise on ways to incorporate forgiveness in your marriage.
5) At the end of the day make a journal entry here on your observations and major takeaways.

_____

_____

_____

_____

_____

_____

_____

_____

_____

_____

_____

_____

Saturday: Divorce

"Therefore, what God has joined together,
let no one separate."
Mark 10:2-9

If after these 90 days you are still considering divorcing your wife or husband, it is a bad idea and you should not do it. Refrian from it because the consequences are devastating on both the husband and wife and the children. Let the following people share their experiences with you;

"Divorce is never a nice thing, but it's very easy to
take family for granted, and when there's a divorce,
you don't take things for granted so much."
Ivanka Trump

"My wife Mary and I have been married for forty-seven years and
not once have we had an argument serious enough to consider
divorce; murder, yes, but divorce, never."
Jack Benny

Some Pharisees came and tested him by asking, "Is it lawful for a man to divorce his wife?"

"What did Moses command you?" he replied.

They said, "Moses permitted a man to write a certificate of divorce and send her away."

*"It was because your hearts were hard that Moses wrote you this law,"
Jesus replied. "But at the beginning of creation God 'made them male
and female.' 'For this reason, a man will leave his father and mother
and be united to his wife, and the two will become one flesh.' So they are
no longer two, but one flesh. Therefore, what God has joined together, let
no one separate." Mark 10:2-9 New International Version (NIV)*

*"I'm going through a divorce now. This is the second one, and like baseball,
I'm not going to get three strikes. I've been living by myself for five years
and I'm very comfortable. I can play my guitar when I want to."* Buddy
Guy

*"In every marriage more than a week old, there are grounds for divorce.
The trick is to find, and continue to find, grounds for marriage."
Robert Anderson*

*"There's nothing like a family crisis, especially a divorce,
to force a person to re-evaluate his life."
Michael Douglas*

*"It's not only moving that creates new starting points. Sometimes all
it takes is a subtle shift in perspective, an opening of the mind, an
intentional pause and reset, or a new route to start to see
new options and new possibilities."
Kristin Armstrong*

Daily to do list

1) Read your why to each other.
2) Read the short daily devotional and meditate
3) Go out and exercise together
4) Focus on forgiveness and what that means to you and your
   relationship. Challenge each other during your exercise on
   ways to incorporate forgiveness in your marriage.

5) At the end of the day make a journal entry here on your
   observations and major takeaways.

_____

_____

_____

_____

_____

_____

_____

_____

_____

_____

_____

_____

_____

_____

_____

_____

_____

_____

_____

_____

What Is Next?

Congratulations for completing this 90-day exercise challenge! Both of you have shown a level of commitment and dedication that is scare among many couples and we want to celebrate it with you. Send us an email at 90daysexercisechallenge@gmail.com for a surprise gift for both of you. We are so proud of your grit, tenacity, and perseverance in completing this challenge. You have joined and exclusive club of finishers and not quitters and by now you can testify firsthand of the benefits and power of exercising together. In the beginning you might not have known what to expect but you took the challenge anyway and went ahead with the program and now you have practical evidence of the joy of regular exercise with your husband or wife.

As you can testify, it was not an easy journey, and nothing was handed to you on a gold platter. You literally had to push yourself to get through this. Now that you are done you may be wondering about what to do next. That is a good place to be in and we are hoping that you will stay there until you come up with something tangible to do. While you are contemplating on what to do, we suggest that you think about the following;

1) Your marriage and what role exercising together is going to play in it from this point forward. Nobody discovers gold or diamonds and walks, they unfailing take the next logical move, that is establish a mine to exploit the diamonds and gold. We believe that you have discovered something that is more than silver and gold and greater than diamonds. Because without good health all the diamonds, silver and gold in the world will be useless to you. You have found the greatest treasure; therefore, develop it and you will eat its

fruits until the end of your lives. In short make exercising regularly, a part of your marriage. You can get another manual and start the process all over and do it again and again. You should always be getting out of a 90-day exercise challenge or getting into one. If you have established the habit you may not need to use the manual, but if the manual will help guide you on the journey then uses it. It is also your right not to do it, but know you cannot escape the negative consequences

2) You were taking notes bring the 90 days and recorded some deep insights about you and your marriage. Some of what you found was surprising and you may be wondering what to do with it. We believe that we are blessed to be a blessing and now is your opportunity to bless others with the treasures that your discovered during your own journey. There are many people who need inspiration and motivation to get their lives and marriages back on track. We can help you do this. Contact us at 90daysexercisechallenge@gmail.com for how to go about this. We are looking forward to working with you and making things better for other people.

3) You have to document your experience during the 90 days challenge and help is available for you to do that. It is possible to make an audio documentation, video documentation or write a book. Yes write a book. If you want to pursue any of these possibilities let is here from you 90daysexercisechallenge@gmail.com.

One last thing!

There is marriage feast with the Lamb that is coming to wards the end of age and will last forever. The Bridegroom is the Alpha and Omega, Jesus Christ the Son of God and we the church are his bride and we have to get ready for this glories marriage and eternal feast. It will be unfair to write about one way to make our earthly marriages work well, but not tell you about the eternal marriage feast. No matter who strong, exciting and enjoyable your marriage is, it peal in comparison to what is being prepared for those who are prepared to meet the Lamb of God when He comes at the end of age.

However, as it is written, *"What no eye has seen, what no ear has heard, and what no human mind has conceived—the things God has prepared for those who love him."* 1 Corinthians 2:9 New International Version (NIV)

This great marriage feast is being prepared for a prepared bride and we are going to share with you how to be prepared.

Before we share how to prepare for this marriage feast of the lamb, it is important to take a quick look at the first marriage that was established by God himself and what happened to it that has brought us to this point of pain, broken relationships, and death.

When God created Adam the first man and placed in the garden of Eden, Adam was lonely, so God created Eve to be his companion. The world of the man was completed when Eve was presented to him thereby establishing the first marriage. There was fellowship between Adam and his wife eve and God until something terrible happened.

God had instructed Adam eat of all the fruits in the garden of Eden but prohibited them not to eat of one particular tree located in the center of the garden. In fact, the instruction stipulated that the day they ate of the tree of the knowledge of good and evil they will die.

One day the serpent (devil) showed up and deceived Eve to eat the forbidden fruit by lying to her that God was disingenuous and restrictive. The devil told Eve that she would become like God when she eats the fruit. Eve fell for this lie, ate the fruit, and gave it to Adam who also ate. Immediately both of them ate the fruit it dawned on them that they were naked. They became ashamed and hid when God showed up. As part of their punishment, God drove them out of the garden of Eden.

You and I are descendants of Adam and Eve, and their act of disobedience resulted in SIN, which signifies the broken relationship between us and God. The following Bible verse in Romans clearly talks about our sin

> *"For all have sinned and fall short of the glory of God."*
> *Romans 3:23*

According to this verse, ALL have sinned including you and me. Nobody is exempted including you. Let me share with you why the issue of sin is troublesome and should be addressed as soon as possible.

> *Sin has a wage, and this wage is not good. Let us*
> *look what the following Bible verse says, "For the*
> *wages of sin is death, but the gift of God is eternal*
> *life in Christ Jesus our Lord."*
> *Romans 6:23*

There is a wage for sin, and that wage is death. We know that death simply means separation. When a loved one dies, we no longer see them because they are separated from us. Likewise, the death that this verse of scripture is referring to is both physical and spiritual. We are separated from God now and if we are not reconciled, we will be separated from God forever and will spend eternity in the pit of hell. This is a place of suffering and torment that is being prepared for the devil and the other fallen angels, and God does not intend for anybody to go there, but if we do not deal with the issue of sin, we will go there when we die the first death.

When it comes to the first death, the following Bible verse clearly states emphatically that it is an appointment, and nobody is exempted from it,

"And as it is appointed unto men once to die,
but after this the judgment."
Hebrews 9:27

According to this verse, death is inevitable, but it is not the END. Everybody including you and me will be judged after we die. This implies that life continues after we transition out of this life. Therefore, it is crucial to prepare for this judgment by the righteous judge who will reward us based on how we lived our lives on earth. The good news is that it is you can know the outcome of the judgment while on earth.

Throughout human history, the gravity of sin and the consciousness of the impending doom has motivated people to do all within their power to resolve this problem to the best of their ability. Many have resorted to being good, religious, ethical, morally pious. Unfortunately, none of these efforts if good enough based on the following scriptures.

"All of us have become like one who is unclean, and all our righteous acts
are like filthy rags; we all shrivel up like a leaf, and like the wind, our
sins sweep us away." Isaiah 64:6

"As Jesus started on his way, a man ran up to him and fell on his knees
before him. 'Good teacher,' he asked, 'what must I do to inherit eternal
life?' 'Why do you call me good?' Jesus answered. 'No one is good –
except God alone. You know the commandments: Do not murder, do
not commit adultery, do not steal, do not give false testimony, do not
defraud, honor your father and mother.' 'Teacher,' he declared, 'all these
I have kept since I was a boy.' Jesus looked at him and loved him. 'One
thing you lack,' he said. 'Go, sell everything you have and give to the
poor, and you will have treasure in heaven. Then come, follow me.' At
this, the man's face fell. He went away sad, because he had great wealth."
Mark 10:17-22

The scripture above describes an eye-opening encounter between Jesus Christ and a rich young ruler as described by another Gospel writer. Based on today's moral standards, this man was "good" and did not need any savior and will have eternal life because he was keeping all the ten commandments. This was a man that was doing all the right things but was aware of his need for eternal life. His question for answers brought him to Jesus Christ, and he enquired about what it will take to get eternal life. In order words what must he do to get into heaven and live with God forever?

When Jesus Christ mentioned keeping the ten commandments, the man's response showed that he had that covered. But Jesus was up to something; it is not what you do that will save you, it is what you believe that matters. That is why Jesus Christ instructed him to do something that the man could not do. Jesus said, 'Go, sell everything you have and give to the poor, and you will have treasure in heaven. Then come, follow me." This was too much for the man to do and he went away sad because he had too much wealth.

The issue that Jesus was pointing at here is a heart issue. The man's wealth was more important than God, that is why he could not part with his wealth. If this man understood that the streets of heaven are made up of God and that there is no more crying, sickness, or death in heaven, he would have easily given up the momentary temporal wealth on earth for the eternal.

But this man could not because his focus was on the earthly, the temporal and what he could do. You may be thinking that I am good and have never harmed anybody and can earn eternal life. You are mistaken

"For it is by grace you have been saved, through faith—and this is not from yourselves, it is the gift of God— not by works, so that no one can boast."
Ephesians 2:8

So far it has been demonstrated All have sinned including you and me and that your works are not good enough to save you and that there is nothing that you can do to earn God's forgiveness and acceptance. Where does this leave us? Is there any hope? What should you do to obtain eternal life?

"Very truly I tell you, whoever hears my word and believes him who sent me has eternal life and will not be judged but has crossed over from death to life."
John 5:24

"But as many as received Him, to them gave the power to become the sons of God, even to them that believe on his name."
John 1:12.

All you need is to believe in Jesus Christ, and you will be saved. When you look at the verb tenses in the versed, you realized that has eternal life means:

Firstly, are having eternal life right now and is not something that you have to die to figure out.

Secondly, "crossed over from death to life," is in the past tense, it implies that you have crossed, it is a done deal the death that sin brings is not going to impact you, it is in the past because you have crossed over.

Thirdly, will not be a judge is referring to the future, this implies that the judgment that sins brings will not impact you now and in the future. Praise God for this assurance.

You may be wondering how to believe or what is it that you are believing, well consider the following.

"But what does it say? "The word is near you, in your mouth and in your heart" (that is, the word of faith which we preach): that if you confess with your mouth the Lord Jesus and believe in your heart that God has raised Him from the dead, you will be saved. For with the heart one believes unto righteousness, and with the mouth confession is made unto salvation. For the Scripture says, "Whoever believes on Him will not be put to shame." For there is no distinction between Jew and Greek, for the same Lord over all is rich to all who call upon Him."
Romans 10:8-12

The word has been presented to you, with the intention of showing how to become reconciled to God so that you can participate in the grand marriage at the end of age with the Son of God and and all you must is

1) Acknowledge that you are a sinner and that you are not good enough and your good works cannot save you
2) Confess your sins to God and ask Him to forgive your sins. Then repent of your sins. This implies that you make a U-turn and start moving towards God instead away from Him
3) Invite Jesus Christ to come into your heart and become your Lord, Savior, and Master.

You can say the following prayer with me or in your own words, but make sure that the prayer contains the three points listed above.

Prayer

Dear heavenly father, I have heard your word, and it has revealed to me that I am a sinner. I am sorry for my sins, and I ask you to forgive me. Give me the gift of eternal life and let me name be written in the Lamb's book of life. I invited Jesus Christ to come into my life and be my personal Lord, savior, and master. I believe that Jesus died on the cross because of my sins and his blood has cleansed me from all my sins. I confess with my mouth that God raised Jesus Christ from the dead and now He is seated at the right-hand side of God the Father and will judge the living and the dead. But I have crossed over from death to life and will no longer be judge because of what Jesus Christ has done for me. Thank you, Lord. In Jesus name, I pray AMEN!

If you prayed this prayer from your heart, you are now a born-again child of God, and I want to be the first person to welcome you into the kingdom of God and congratulate for making the most crucial decisions of your life. If you need more help, make your request through this email; eternalkingdom101@gmail.com.

Pass It On

We are not going to ask of you something that you cannot do, because that will be unfair. When you eat in a good restaurant or find a good deal your first reaction is to think of somebody love that can benefit as well. You do not allow your lack of sells training to prevent you from telling your loved ones that there is good food down the street or that there is a good deal that will save them some money. The excitement and love you have prompts and compels you to share with others. This has been an amazing journey for you have learned a lot and now the charge we have for you is to simply pass it on. You have the resources and should get one other couple to go through what you and your husband or wife have. If you do not share with them who will? Those close to you are looking up to you and some might have already asked you questions, you do not need to be an expert to answer these questions. All you need to do is share your own experiences and if in doubt email us and call.

Authors' Biographies

Dr. Eric Tangumonkem

Dr. Eric Tangumonkem was born and raised in Cameroon and migrated to the United States of America in 2002. He holds degrees in geology, earth sciences, and geosciences and is a professor of environmental missions at Missional University. Eric is an author and speaker on a mission to inspire, equip, and motivate people to find, pursue, and possess their God-given purpose. He is the co-founder and president of Equipping of the Saints International Ministries. Eric lives with his wife and five children in Richardson, Texas. Follow him on Twitter,

@DrTangumonkem, and Facebook, drtangumonkem.

Elizabeth Tayem

Elizabeth Tayem is an author, speaker, self-motivated, articulate, and value driven, Early Childhood Intervention Specialist with extensive training in developmental screening assessments and related research. She graduated with an Associate of applied Science in Child Development (Magna cum Laude) from Colin College and obtained a Bachelor's degree in Psychology and a minor in Child Learning and Development from the University of Texas at Dallas and a Master's in Developmental Psychology with emphasis in Human Development and Early Childhood Disorder from the University of Texas at Dallas. She also has extensive experience working with children and families in clinical settings, hospital, day-care, preschool and grade school and is the founder and director of Tayem Care with Passion that offers child care to children from 0-5 years old and Tayem Parenting Consulting that equips parents of children from 0-12 years on how to be effective and efficient parents.

She is a mother of five beautiful God given children and is an advocate of heling through nutrition and exercise. Her holistic approach has been the subject of most of her talks, research and writing.

It is unfortunate that everything these days is hijacked and turned into a political weapon. Those who hate president Trump do not want to ask the right questions. How will open boarders help everybody? How will lawlessness benefit all of us? Is it fair that you drive above the speed limit and have to pay a fine and those who are here illegally are reward for breaking immigration law? As long as the laws are in the books they must be enforced, if we do not like the laws, they should be changed.

Printed in Dunstable, United Kingdom